Making the Prostate Therapy Decision

Also by Jeff Baggish:

How Your Immune System Works

Making the Prostate Therapy Decision

Jeff Baggish, M.D.

Foreword by Mark R. Silk, M.D.

Lowell House
Los Angeles

Contemporary Books
Chicago

Library of Congress Cataloging-in-Publication Data

Baggish, Jeff.
  Making the prostate therapy decision / by Jeff Baggish; foreword by Mark
Silk.
    p. cm.
  Includes bibliographical references and index.
  ISBN 1-56565-433-1
  1. Prostate—Popular works. I. Title
  RC899.B33 1995
  616.6'5—dc20   95-14199

Requests for such permissions should be addressed to:
Lowell House
2029 Century Park East, Suite 3290
Los Angeles, CA 90067

Lowell House books can be purchased at special discounts
when ordered in bulk for premiums and special sales.
Contact Department JH at the address above.

Publisher: Jack Artenstein
General Manager, Lowell House Adult: Bud Sperry
Text design: Robert S. Tinnon Design
Illustrations © 1995 Elizabeth Weadon Massari

Manufactured in the United States of America
10 9 8 7 6 5 4 3 2 1

This book is dedicated to my father, Dr. Michael S. Baggish, who has been my mentor, role model, inspiration, and friend since the day I was born.

CONTENTS

FOREWORD

If someone were to ask me to select a single word to describe the current environment surrounding the topic of prostate cancer, it would be *controversial*. These days, it's hard to pick up a newspaper or turn on the television without seeing something about the diagnosis and treatment of this disease. Tests like prostate-specific antigen (PSA) and transrectal ultrasound (TRUS), which didn't even exist a few short years ago, are now used routinely and receive a lot of media coverage. The only problem is that doctors who treat prostate cancer can't agree amongst themselves about when and how best to utilize these new tools. New treatment strategies and surgical techniques seem to be popping up on an almost daily basis, but there are almost as many different views about which treatment is best as there are people forming opinions. How is news of these cutting-edge developments of any use to the patient if the experts themselves can't agree on anything?

Fortunately, Jeff Baggish has written *Making the Prostate Therapy Decision* to help you sift through all the confusion and arm yourself with the information you need to make intelligent decisions about your health. Too many books about prostate disease are written by specialists whose advice is biased by their fields of interest. Urologists typically lean toward surgery, while oncologists usually favor radiation therapy. Dr. Baggish, on the other hand, presents a fair and balanced assessment of all the treatment options, including the choice not to treat, so that you, the prostate cancer patient, can be the one making these important decisions.

Not only is *Making the Prostate Therapy Decision* an unbiased source of information, but a comprehensive one as well. Jeff Baggish really has done his research here, and nothing important is left out. At the same time, nothing irrelevant is included. Dr. Baggish presents only the cold, hard facts that you need to know without wasting your time on the excess "fluff" that fills the pages of so many other books on this subject.

Facts presented in an unbiased, comprehensive manner won't help you if you can't understand the language. This is where Dr. Baggish's talents really come into play. In the thirty-plus years that I've known Jeff, I've always been impressed by his love of teaching and the ease with which he can explain complex topics to people who have had no medical training. *Making the Prostate Therapy Decision* is a shining example of this ability. No experience with medical terminology whatsoever is necessary in order for you to fully understand and enjoy this book.

As you read this book, you will learn about prostate disease in a logical, step-by-step manner. Chapters 1 and 2 explain the basics about normal and abnormal prostate anatomy and function. Chapters 3 and 4 then cover the various methods by which physicians can identify cancer of the prostate before it becomes a problem. The subsequent four chapters present everything that you'll need to know about the various forms of prostate cancer treatment, including the no-treatment school of thought that has become increasingly popular in recent years. Chapter 9 deals with the new and exciting area of prostate cancer prevention strategies, while chapter 10 is devoted to the extremely important psychological issues that affect not only men, but their loved ones as well. Finally, chapters

11 and 12 discuss benign enlargement of the prostate (BPH), a condition that is far less dangerous than prostate cancer, but far more common and with far more uncomfortable symptoms.

Making the Prostate Therapy Decision is informative, accurate, comprehensive, unbiased, and easy to understand. If you buy only one book about prostate disease, this should be it!

MARK R. SILK, M.D.
Assistant Professor of Urology
University of Connecticut
School of Medicine
Farmington, CT

ILLUSTRATIONS

TABLES

ACKNOWLEDGMENTS

I will be forever grateful to Dr. Mark Silk for providing technical review and for writing the foreword to this book. I would never have been able to complete this project without his expert assistance.

I also wish to extend my thanks to my editor, Bud Sperry, and managing editor, Maria Magallanes, and all of the folks at RGA Lowell House.

Making the Prostate Therapy Decision

What Is the Prostate Gland?

Given the astounding degree of technologic sophistication existing in medical science today, it is surprising that there is still no satisfactory answer to the question, "What is the prostate and what does it do?" The prostate is like the appendix: it is not essential for life and its exact function is difficult to define. In fact, as with your appendix, you probably never thought about it—until something went wrong.

While general understanding of the prostate is less than perfect, if you have a disease like prostate cancer or benign prostatic hyperplasia, you should know as much as possible about the architecture and function of this gland to make an informed therapy decision. This chapter covers basic prostatic anatomy and physiology.

What Is the Prostate?

The prostate is the largest of the four accessory glands of the male reproductive system; the others are the seminal vesicles, the bulbourethral (Cowper's) glands, and the prostatic utricle (Table 1.1). The prostate weighs about ¾ ounce and is about the size of a walnut. Its dimensions are about ¾ inch thick, 1¼ inches long, and 1½ inches wide. Its main function is to produce prostatic fluid, one of several substances that compose semen.

Table 1.1
Accessory Glands of the Male Reproductive System

1. Prostate
2. Seminal Vesicles
3. Bulbourethral (Cowper's) Glands
4. Prostatic Utricle

The cells that secrete prostatic fluid are arranged into 30 to 50 discrete glandular units, or acini, within the prostate. The fluid produced by these glands drains into 15 to 30 independent excretory ducts, which lead to the urethra, the tube that carries semen (and urine) outside the body. That part of the prostate where the ducts empty into the urethra is a "bump" of tissue called the verumontanum, or colliculus seminalis, protruding from the back wall of the urethra like a tiny volcano.

The fluid-secreting acini are tightly encased within a mass of muscular and fibrous tissue that makes up the rest of the prostate organ. The entire prostate is surrounded by a thick fibrous capsule, and a number of fibrous walls, or septa, fan out from the verumontanum (on the inside) to the capsule (on the outside), dividing the prostate into separate partitions. The capsule squeezes fluid out of the prostate during ejaculation.

Where Is the Prostate in Relation to Other Organs?

The prostate is directly beneath the bladder, sandwiched between the front wall of the pelvis and the rectum (Figure 1.1). As the urethra carries urine out of the bladder, it

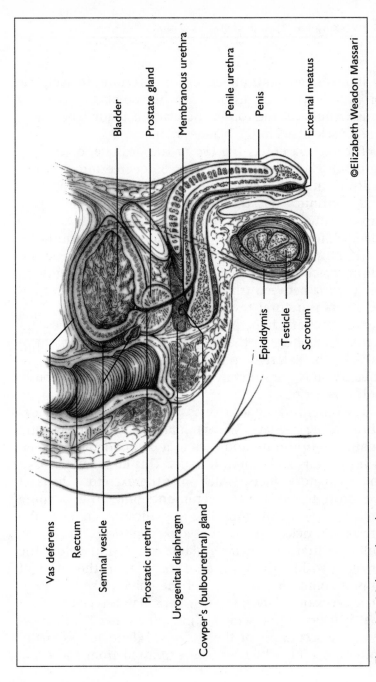

Vas deferens

Rectum

Seminal vesicle

Prostatic urethra

Urogenital diaphragm

Cowper's (bulbourethral) gland

Bladder

Prostate gland

Membranous urethra

Penile urethra

Penis

External meatus

Epididymis

Testicle

Scrotum

©Elizabeth Weadon Massari

Figure 1.1: Male genitourinary anatomy

is immediately surrounded by the prostate. In fact, the prostate is so closely associated with the bladder that the muscle fibers at the top of the gland actually blend with the muscle fibers in the bladder wall.

The urethra enters the top of the prostate, dives deep into the gland, takes an abrupt 35-degree forward turn halfway through (where the verumontanum is located), and continues out through the bottom of the organ. Prostate muscle fibers surround the urethra as it exits the bladder, forming the internal or preprostatic sphincter. This sphincter prevents semen from flowing backward during ejaculation, and also keeps urine from lingering in the urethra between trips to the bathroom. Men who undergo transurethral resection of the prostate (TURP) for benign prostatic hyperplasia (BPH) typically lose these internal sphincters in the process. An additional band of muscle, the external sphincter, is located farther downstream and is the structure that allows you to consciously hold your urine.

The other three male accessory glands are in close proximity to the prostate. The seminal vesicles are above and behind the prostate and secrete a component of semen rich in sugars and other nutrients. This fluid empties into the ejaculatory ducts, which, like the excretory ducts of the prostate, end at the verumontanum. Also opening onto the verumontanum, like the volcano's crater, is the prostatic utricle, a small embryologic leftover. Finally, the bulbourethral or Cowper's glands are found below the prostate within the urogenital diaphragm, the sheet of muscle composing the floor of the pelvis. Like the other male accessory glands, the Cowper's glands secrete a fluid that helps compose semen. Unlike the other fluids, however, the secretions of the Cowper's glands occasionally contain sperm, which can be expressed from the penis even before ejaculation occurs, which is why "premature withdrawal" is an ineffective birth control method.

Now let's tie everything together and trace the path of sperm and semen from start to finish. Sperm are formed within the seminiferous tubules of the testes. They exit the testes through another collection of tubes called the epididymus and enter the main sperm-carrying duct, the vas deferens. The vas deferens is severed in a vasectomy, the surgical procedure that blocks the route sperm use to reach the penis. The vas carries sperm the length of the scrotum and into the pelvis, where it widens into the ampulla before emptying into the ejaculatory ducts behind the prostate. We already know the seminal vesicles also empty into the ejaculatory ducts. The ejaculatory ducts, in turn, enter the back of the prostate and open into the urethra just below the prostatic utricle's opening on the verumontanum; the verumontanum itself is flanked by the many openings of the excretory ducts of the prostate.

The segment of the urethra contained within the prostate, the prostatic urethra, leads to the urogenital diaphragm, at which point it becomes the membranous urethra, and into the penis, where it is called the penile urethra. The final ingredient of semen, produced by the Cowper's glands, empties into the penile urethra. Sperm and semen then exit the penis through the external meatus.

Do Some Regions of the Prostate Differ from Others?

As it travels the length of the prostate, the urethra divides the gland into two portions (see Figure 1.2). The front, or anterior, portion is composed largely of fibrous tissue and muscle. The glandular units of the prostate are found

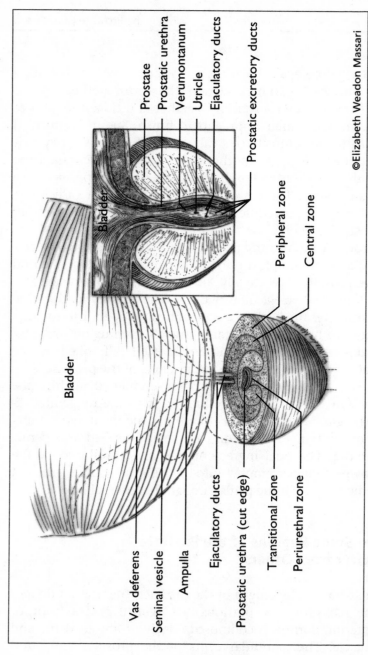

Figure 1.2: Zones of the prostate.

Prostate
Prostatic urethra
Verumontanum
Utricle
Ejaculatory ducts
Prostatic excretory ducts

Bladder

©Elizabeth Weadon Massari

Peripheral zone
Central zone

Bladder

Vas deferens
Seminal vesicle
Ampulla
Ejaculatory ducts
Prostatic urethra (cut edge)
Transitional zone
Periurethral zone

Table 1.2
Zones of the Prostate

1. Peripheral Zone (approx. 65–75%)
2. Central Zone (approx. 20–25%)
3. Transition Zone (approx. 5–10%)
4. Periurethral Zone (approx. 1%)

mostly in the rear, or posterior, portion. This way of dividing the prostate is not very useful, however, when discussing the function of the organ and the diseases that affect it.

Most doctors today like to split the prostate into four distinct areas with respect to microscopic anatomy and excretory duct drainage. These four regions are the peripheral zone, comprising 65–75 percent of the gland, the central zone, occupying 20–25 percent of the prostate, the transition zone, making up 5–10 percent of the prostate, and the periurethral zone, containing about 1 percent of the prostatic tissue (Table 1.2).

The central zone of the prostate surrounds the ejaculatory ducts as they enter the back of the gland and head toward the verumontanum. The prostatic excretory ducts residing in the central zone also empty at the verumontanum near the openings for the ejaculatory ducts. The glandular units within the central zone tend to be larger and more irregular than those in the peripheral zone, the excretory ducts draining them branch more elaborately than peripheral zone ducts, and the muscular tissue encasing them is more densely packed than that of the peripheral zone. Only 8 percent of prostate cancers develop in the central zone.

As the name implies, peripheral zone tissue is situated toward the outer aspect of the prostate. Excretory ducts within this region empty into the urethra farther downstream than those of the central zone. The peripheral zone is typified by glands that are smaller and more uniform than those of the central zone, with a simpler excretory duct system and looser muscular tissue. The most significant characteristic of the peripheral zone, however, is that it is the preferred site for the development of prostate cancer; approximately 72 percent of all cases arise here.

The preferred site for benign prostatic hyperplasia (BPH), on the other hand, is the transition zone. This region of the prostate extends outward in winglike fashion from the area of the internal urethral sphincter and, in 20 percent of cases, is less likely to become cancerous than the peripheral zone. That the transition zone is so close to the urethra is significant when BPH occurs, because the growth eventually obstructs urine flow out of the bladder.

The final region of the prostate is the periurethral zone, the narrow strip of tissue contained within the internal sphincter itself. As with the transition zone, BPH also develops in the periurethral zone.

Do Glandular Units Differ from Zone to Zone?

Yes. The glands of the peripheral zone, where prostate cancer usually arises, are called main prostatic glands. BPH occurs in the smaller mucosal glands of the transition and periurethral zones. These glands are surrounded by a ring of yet another intermediate-sized gland type, the submucosal glands (Table 1.3). Each gland type has its own system of excretory ducts to drain the fluid they produce.

Table 1.3
Prostate Gland Types

1. Main Prostatic Glands: Large. Peripheral zone.
2. Mucosal Glands: Small. Transition and Periurethral zones.
3. Submucosal Glands: Intermediate. Ring around mucosal glands.

The fluid-manufacturing cells of the various prostatic glands all share a dependence on the male hormone testosterone, produced by the Leydig cells of the testes, for normal growth and development. When the testosterone supply is interrupted by castration, whether from drugs or surgery, the cells of the prostate glands shrink and lose their ability to secrete prostatic fluid. You may wonder why anyone would want to do that, but it is a desirable result if the cells happen to be cancerous, which explains the rationale behind the use of castration to treat advanced prostate cancer.

What Is Contained in Prostatic Fluid?

Prostatic fluid is a thin, milky secretion containing many ingredients, among them citric acid, calcium, zinc, and a variety of enzymes (Table 1.4). Undoubtedly, the most important of the enzymes is acid phosphatase, because increased blood levels of this chemical have, until recently, been essential in diagnosing and treating prostate cancer. The main drawback of using acid phosphatase levels to diagnose cancer of the prostate is that the enzyme is also

---

Table 1.4
Partial List of Prostatic Fluid Contents

1. Citric acid
2. Calcium
3. Zinc
4. Acid phosphatase
5. Alkaline phosphatase
6. Fibrinolysin
7. Sialic acid
8. Spermine
9. Prostaglandin
10. Amylase
11. Fibrinogenase
12. Aminopeptidase
13. Transaminase
14. β-glucuronidase
15. Diastase

---

used to diagnose diseases of other organs, such as the liver, pancreas, lungs, intestines, white blood cells, and bone, and is thus not entirely specific for prostate disease. Its usefulness as a prostate diagnostic tool has largely been replaced by the discovery of prostate-specific antigen (PSA), which, as its name implies, appears nowhere but in the prostate. PSA is covered in greater detail in chapter 4.

Besides adding volume to semen, prostatic fluid serves another important function. Its alkaline quality helps neutralize the acidity of vaginal fluid during intercourse. Acidity can inhibit the fertilizing ability of sperm, so neutralizing this hostile environment with prostatic fluid increases a sperm's chances of surviving and reaching its destination.

Sometimes prostatic fluid that lingers within the glands and ducts can solidify into tiny "beads" called prostatic concretions, or *corpora amylacea*. Concretion formation is a normal occurrence, and the number of concretions contained within the prostate increases as you age. Small concretions typically pass into the semen without difficulty, while larger ones may become lodged within a gland or excretory duct. Prostatic concretions frequently become hardened with calcium, at which point they are referred to as calculi, or stones.

Now that you know all about how the prostate functions normally, you're ready to find out what happens when things go wrong. Chapter 2 deals with cancer of the prostate.

Chapter 2

What Is Prostate Cancer?

We are all familiar with the term *cancer* and use it freely in writing and conversation. But if someone were to ask you to define cancer, you would probably have a tough time doing so. You could picture the disorder in your mind and the answer might dangle at the tip of your tongue, but a clear-cut, dictionary-type description would escape you. This chapter is about cancer.

First let's define *neoplasm*, a new and abnormal growth or tumor that can affect any organ in the body. It begins as a single cell that becomes abnormal, then multiplies at the expense of the normal cells surrounding it. Neoplasms are classified as benign or malignant depending upon their tendency to metastasize, or spread, to other organs. A benign tumor, although it may grow to considerable size, does not invade other structures. A malignant neoplasm, on the other hand, if left untreated, has the potential to metastasize to other parts of the body. Cancer is the term most of us use when referring to malignant neoplasms.

Cancer that affects our skeletal building blocks, such as bone, muscle, cartilage, and fibrous tissue, is called sarcoma. Cancer that arises in visceral organs like the lung, breast, colon, and prostate is referred to as *carcinoma*. Therefore, we can define carcinoma of the prostate as a new growth of abnormal cells that thrives at the expense of the rest of the organ, and if left untreated, can metastasize to other parts of the body.

How Common Is Prostate Cancer?

To understand the statistics of any disease, first you must become familiar with the terms *incidence, prevalence*, and *mortality*. Imagine a giant bubble gum machine partially filled with gumballs, each piece representing a man who has prostate cancer. The number of gumballs in the machine would equal the total number of cases, or prevalence, of prostate cancer in the population. Now, imagine someone has removed the machine lid and is slowly adding gumballs to those already present. The number of new gumballs added during a particular period would reflect the number of new cases, or incidence, of prostate cancer. As new cases are added to the existing pool of prostate cancer in the community, a certain number of men leave the pool either by dying from the disease (mortality) or by being cured. Add that to your gumball machine example by picturing someone removing gumballs from the bottom of the machine. Incidence has the effect of increasing the prevalence of a disease, while mortality and cure have the opposite effect, and both influences occur simultaneously.

Carcinoma of the prostate is the most common type of cancer in American men. It is estimated that prostate cancer has a prevalence of 30 percent or more among men over 50, which means a third of all men over 50 have some degree of cancer in their prostates, whether or not they know it. This prevalence increases with age until more than half of all men in their eighties have prostate cancer.

The incidence of prostate cancer is also higher than for any other cancer in men. Over 130,000 new cases of the disease are diagnosed each year, and because men are living longer and methods of early detection are improving, the incidence is increasing steadily. Today, prostate cancer represents 23 percent of all new cancers in men.

The mortality from prostate cancer is exceeded only by lung cancer and represents 12 percent of all male cancer deaths. At over 35,000 deaths each year in the U.S., prostate cancer claims a life every 15 minutes. Among black men the mortality is twice that of white men, despite the fact that the incidences within the two groups are the same. However, prostate carcinomas in black men are usually more aggressive and rapid-growing. Overall, any male who is born in the U.S. has a 9–13 percent chance of developing prostate cancer sometime during his life and a 2½–3 percent chance of dying from it.

Are Some Men More Likely Than Others to Get Prostate Cancer?

Considerable research has focused on identifying risk factors for prostate cancer, those elements that make a person likelier to acquire the disease. Many potential culprits have been investigated, but only a few have consistently been, or consistently *not* been, associated with increased risk of developing prostate carcinoma. The cause of the disease remains unknown.

Studies have revealed only two scenarios that invariably increase a man's risk of developing prostate cancer: being a farmer and having one or more first-degree relatives (a father or brother) with the disease. No one is quite sure why farmers have a higher rate of prostate cancer than the general population, but they do. The family history connection is also quite clear. If your father or brother has prostate cancer, you have two to three times greater risk of developing the disease than someone who doesn't have an affected relative; having *two* first-degree relatives makes it *five* times likelier you will get it.

Other factors definitely *do not* increase your risk of developing prostate cancer. No association exists between carcinoma of prostate and radiation exposure, alcohol consumption, or tobacco smoking, although these entities are risk factors for other diseases. Smoking, for example, has consistently been linked to heart disease, emphysema, lung cancer, and a host of other health problems. Many other potential prostate risk factors have been studied and have yielded equivocal results. The connection between prostate cancer and a man's number of sexual partners, his occupation (except farmer), viral infections, benign prostatic hyperplasia (BPH), vasectomy, or exposure to various chemicals varies depending on whose data you read. Special relationships do exist between prostate cancer and sunlight, vitamin D, dietary fat, and exercise, and we'll discuss those in chapter 9.

We already know that being black does not place a man at greater risk of getting prostate cancer, but blacks tend to develop the disease at an earlier age than whites so their cancer is usually more advanced when diagnosed. Black men are more likely to die of prostate carcinoma than white men.

In the previous chapter, we mentioned a correlation between the male hormone testosterone and the growth of prostate cells, whether or not they are cancerous. It has long been known that eunuchs, men who were castrated before the onset of puberty, do not get prostate cancer. However, while male hormone can enhance the growth of a prostate tumor, most scientists agree it does not cause cancer. In addition, it does not appear that a man's blood level of testosterone has anything to do with his risk of acquiring prostate carcinoma.

Prostate cancer is disproportionately represented in certain parts of the world. Sweden and the United States have the highest incidences. European countries like Spain, France, and Italy hover around the middle of the list. The lowest prostate cancer rates are found in Asian countries like China, Japan, and Singapore, but Asians in the U.S. have a significantly higher incidence of prostate carcinoma than Asians in Asia; the same is true of blacks in the U.S. versus blacks in Africa. This suggests that the variation in cancer rates among the different nationalities is not only a result of genetics, but environmental factors as well.

Are There Different Types of Prostate Cancer?

Virtually 95 percent of all prostate cancers arise in the acini (glandular units) of the organ. Tumors that develop here are called adenocarcinoma, which means "cancer of the gland." The remaining 5 percent of prostate cancers are of many different types. Some resemble bladder cancer; others are metastases from tumors in other organs. Some begin in the muscle of the gland, others in the excretory ducts. Carcinoma of the ducts is not only more aggressive than adenocarcinoma, but also more difficult to detect early, because it does not secrete significant amounts of prostate-specific antigen (PSA). Fortunately, its occurrence is rare. PSA will be discussed in greater detail in chapter 4.

Are Some Adenocarcinomas More Dangerous Than Others?

The term *grade* is used when referring to the aggressiveness and malignant potential of a tumor cell. The grade of a cancer cell depends on its degree of differentiation, or the closeness with which it resembles the normal cells of the organ. Tumors that are well-differentiated can mimic the function of normal cells and are of a lower grade. Poorly differentiated cancer cells do not look at all like their normal counterparts and are given a higher grade. In general, high-grade cancers are associated with a greater tendency toward metastasis and a poorer prognosis.

Prostate cancer differs from malignancies affecting many other organs, because a variety of grades may be found within a single tumor. Some cells in a prostate tumor may be very aggressive while others in the same tumor may be nonaggressive. The heterogeneous nature of prostate cancer has made it a challenge to predict which tumors will progress rapidly and metastasize and which will remain stable for long periods.

As a way of getting around this problem, most experts have adopted the Gleason grading system when assessing the malignant potential of prostate cancer. In this system, the two groups of cancer cells that occupy the greatest volume within a given tumor are assigned a number from 1 to 5, depending on the differentiation of the cells in each group. Cells with the best possible grade are given a score of 1; those with the poorest degree of differentiation receive a score of 5. The scores of the two regions are added together to produce a Gleason score between 2 and 10. A high Gleason score indicates a more malignant tumor and is thus associated with a worse prognosis than one with a low score. The Gleason system is not the only grading method. Over 40 different grading systems have been used. But the Gleason is the most widely accepted system and the one you are most likely to encounter if you or someone you know develops prostate cancer.

Knowing the Gleason score of a tumor can help a doctor decide which methods of diagnosis and treatment are most appropriate. A high score in a cancer found incidentally during transurethral resection (TURP) for benign prostatic hyperplasia (BPH) or one removed before it has shown obvious signs of extending beyond the gland should prompt further investigation for metastases. High Gleason scores are associated with a greater likelihood of capsule penetration, invasion of the seminal vesicles, and metastases to the lymph nodes, bone, or central nervous system.

The main drawback to grade as a predictor of tumor malignancy is that it is highly subjective. One pathologist might consider a prostate cancer to be high-grade, while another may label the same tumor with an intermediate score. Thus, a Gleason score may not always reflect the true biologic potential of a tumor. Considerable research is devoted currently to finding a better indicator of malignant potential. One of these methods, flow cytometry, is discussed in the next chapter.

Does the Size of the Tumor Matter?

Yes. Grade alone cannot determine what action you should take. Your doctor must also know the stage of the tumor to make an informed therapy decision. Surgery can potentially cure a carcinoma contained entirely within the prostate gland, but obviously it will not help someone whose cancer has spread (metastasized) to other organs.

Prostate cancer can spread along a number of routes. As it grows and pushes through the capsule, it can directly invade the bladder, urethra, or seminal vesicles. Tumor cells can also escape through the lymphatic channels that cleanse and drain the prostate of pollutants. As these cancer cells float downstream, they deposit along the way in the lymph nodes. The lymph nodes of the pelvis are the preferred site, but nodes surrounding the major blood vessels, such as the iliacs and the aorta, also can become involved. Prostate cancer can also metastasize through the bloodstream and invade bones such as the pelvis, vertebrae, or ribs; or visceral organs like the lungs, liver, or adrenal glands.

The staging method most frequently used to classify prostate cancer is the Whitmore-Jewett system, which assigns a stage of A, B, C, or D to a given prostate tumor, depending upon its degree of advancement (Table 2.1). As many as half of all diagnosed prostate cancers are found incidentally in tissue that is removed during a TURP for BPH. In these cases, the physician performs the TURP thinking the prostate harbors only benign disease, because the tumor is too small to be felt during a digital rectal examination (DRE). This stage of early carcinoma is stage A. A larger tumor that can be felt by a doctor performing a DRE is considered stage B. Once a cancer extends beyond the capsule of the prostate, it is labeled stage C tumor. Stage D cancers have metastasized to lymph nodes or other organs.

These stages are divided further into sub-classifications. A stage A tumor found in three or fewer locations within the prostate is called a stage A1 cancer; one with three or more sites (or occupying more than 5 percent of the prostate tissue) is classified as A2. Stage B1N, between stages A2 and B1, is given to cancers that are 1.5 cm (0.6 in.) or less in diameter, confined to one side of the prostate, and completely surrounded by normal tissue. Stage B carcinomas are divided into those that are B1, or

Table 2.1
Whitmore-Jewett Staging System

Stage A1: 1, 2, or 3 areas of well-differentiated tumor
Stage A2: >3 areas of well-differentiated tumor or any quantity of higher grade tumor
Stage B1n: nodule <1.5 cm in diameter, occupying <1 side of prostate, normal tissue on all 4 sides
Stage B1: nodule occupying <1 side of prostate with normal tissue on 3 sides
Stage B2: nodule on both sides of prostate
Stage C1: Penetration through capsule
Stage C2: Extension to seminal vesicles
Stage D1: Metastasis to pelvic lymph nodes
Stage D2: Metastasis to distant sites
Stage D3: Metastatic disease not responsive to hormone therapy

residing in only one side of the gland, and those that are B2, or extending across both sides of the prostate. C1 tumors have extended outside the prostate, while C2 carcinomas have invaded the seminal vesicles. Stage D1 is assigned to cancers that have spread to the lymph nodes of the pelvis, and D2 is the classification for tumors that have metastasized to the bone, distant lymph nodes, or other organs. A new, not yet widely accepted stage of D3 is assigned to cancers that have metastasized and will not respond to hormonal therapy.

A different method called the TNM (tumor, nodes, metastases) system is usually used for staging cancer in organs other than the prostate (Table 2.2). Some physicians use this system in staging prostate cancer as well, but the Whitmore system is used more frequently in the U.S. The

---

Table 2.2
TNM Staging System

Tumor Size:
  T1a: Less than 5% of prostate tissue, cannot be felt
  T1b: More than 5% of prostate tissue, cannot be felt
  T2a: small nodule, less than one side of gland
  T2b: small nodule, one side of gland
  T2c: Involving both sides, confined to prostate
   T3: Penetrates capsule
   T4: Spread to neighboring tissue and organs

Lymph Nodes:
  N1: 1 node, same side as tumor
  N2: multiple nodes or node on opposite side of tumor
  N3: Extensive involvement of pelvic lymph nodes
  N4: Involvement of lymph nodes outside of pelvis

Metastases:
  M0: no metastases
  M1: metastases

(Note: Variations on the TNM Staging System exist.)

TNM method assigns a T number to a tumor that corresponds to its size, an N number indicating whether lymph nodes are involved, and an M number reflecting the presence or absence of metastases.

Neither grade nor stage alone can dictate appropriate therapy for any individual case of prostate cancer. Low-grade tumors can be very large, while small tumors can be highly malignant. Both variables must be taken into account when you and your doctor are deciding on the treament plan that is best for you.

What Are the Symptoms of Prostate Cancer?

Most cancers that are confined to the prostate and are potentially curable cause no symptoms at all, which is why so many men carry cancer within their prostate glands without ever knowing it. By the time the cancer is discovered, it is often too late to remove the entire tumor with surgery alone. As many as 25–35 percent of prostate cancers reach stage C or D by the time they are diagnosed; a number that may be even higher among black patients.

The first objective sign of prostate cancer is usually induration, or hardening, of the gland. Obviously, you cannot touch your own prostate to check for induration, so you must rely on your doctor to discover this important warning sign. That's why a complete annual check-up that includes a digital rectal examination is so important.

If a tumor is allowed to advance beyond the mere induration stage, the first symptoms usually arise because the flow of urine from the bladder is obstructed These symptoms may include any or all of the following: painful urination, difficulty initiating urination, slowing of the urinary stream, dribbling of urine, the sensation of incomplete bladder emptying, increased frequency of urination, and an increased need to urinate at night. Blood in the urine is rare, but can occur. A tumor that encroaches upon the bladder outlet may also cause increased susceptibility to urinary tract infections (UTI). UTIs are common in women, but are quite uncommon in men and often indicate a more significant underlying problem, so any radical changes in your urinary habits should be evaluated by your doctor.

Symptoms arising from metastatic cancer depend on the organ invaded. Lung metastases can cause shortness of breath. Bone metastases can lead to bone pain, especially in the hip or lower back; fractures from an abnormally small degree of force; or compression of the spinal cord, which can lead to pain, weakness, or numbness in the legs. Metastases that are more widespread can cause weight loss, leg swelling, lymph node enlargement, or kidney failure. Curiously, impotence usually is not a symptom of prostate cancer.

Chapter 3

How Is Prostate Cancer Diagnosed and Staged?

To make the right prostate therapy decision, you'll not only need to know whether or not cancer is present, but also the extent to which it has progressed. For example, if a cancer is found to be completely contained within the prostate, removing the organ surgically (prostatectomy) can cure the disease. A tumor that has spread to areas outside of the prostate eliminates surgery from the list of treatment options. This chapter will describe some of the tools a physician can use to diagnose prostate cancer, and also for staging the cancers that are diagnosed.

What Is a Digital Rectal Exam?

The digital rectal examination (DRE) is the simplest, least expensive, most widely available, and probably the most valuable procedure for diagnosing and assessing prostate disease. The DRE can also investigate tumors of the rectum and reveal traces of blood in the stool, which can be an early sign of colon cancer. This procedure is the first step usually taken when examining the prostate and should precede other, more elaborate tests.

The DRE is an examination of the rectum, the last segment of the colon, or large intestine, the organ that carries stool to the outside world. A DRE can and should be performed every year by your regular doctor once you reach a certain age. In preparing you for a DRE, your doctor will ask you either to bend over or to lie on your side with your knees curled up to your chest. He will then insert a lubricated, gloved finger into your rectum and feel for any abnormalities in the size, shape, or consistency of the prostate gland, which lies outside the front rectal wall in the pelvis.

The chief piece of evidence your physician is searching for when he does a DRE is induration of the prostate gland. Induration occurs early in the evolution of prostate cancer and if detected leads the way to more specific diagnostic tests that offer the best chances for successful treatment. However, when induration is subtle, as it often is, then it can be missed by all but the most experienced physicians. Another disadvantage of induration as a diagnostic sign is that it occurs in many situations besides prostate cancer. Prostatic calculi (stones), benign prostatic hyperplasia (BPH), dead prostate tissue, prostate infections, and scar tissue are but a few of the processes that can cause induration of this organ. In fact, 25–50 percent of all men with prostatic induration end up *not* having cancer. Still, it is better to be safe than sorry: all areas of induration should be considered cancerous until proven otherwise.

The DRE itself has several other disadvantages. It is subjective. Its accuracy depends largely upon the technique and skill of the physician performing it. An experienced urologist may be able to detect subtle changes within the prostate and may also be able to roughly estimate the stage of a cancerous prostate. Because rectal exams represent a much smaller portion of an internist's or family practitioner's daily practice, a more obvious change in the prostate might be necessary for a nonspecialist to notice it. Regardless of a physician's degree of experience, a DRE obviously cannot detect the microscopic spread of cancer across the prostatic capsule or metastases into the lymph nodes or bone. In fact, the previous chapter explained that a stage A prostate carcinoma cannot be felt during a DRE, so any cancer detected by DRE must automatically be stage B or higher.

While a DRE cannot detect cancer at its earliest possible stage, it is far superior to the alternative: *not* undergoing a DRE. Therefore, any man over 40 should have an annual DRE as part of his complete check-up. Men with risk factors like those mentioned in the previous chapter should begin routine DREs even sooner. Anyone with suspicious urinary or gastrointestinal symptoms should also have a DRE, regardless of his age.

What Do I Do if My DRE Is Suspicious?

If the doctor feels an abnormal growth within the prostate gland, the obvious next step is to find out if it is cancerous, which is best accomplished by obtaining an actual piece, or biopsy, of the suspicious area, then examining it under a microscope. Like any manipulation of the prostate, a biopsy can cause an artificially high prostate-specific antigen (PSA) level in the blood. The PSA level is important not only in diagnosing and staging prostate cancer, but in determining the success of treatment. Your doctor will want a baseline PSA reading that is as accurate as possible, so he will probably collect that before performing a biopsy. PSA is covered in greater detail in the following chapter.

No biopsy should be ordered unless the doctor has decided the result will influence the choice of treatment. A young, otherwise healthy man whose biopsy is positive for cancer can realistically consider any surgical, radiologic, or hormonal treatment option that is appropriate for his stage of disease. An older man with multiple health problems, on the other hand, is not likely to prolong his life by pursuing aggressive therapy. On the contrary, the risks and side effects of some treatment choices may actually shorten or adversely affect the quality of his remaining life; these men should *not* undergo prostatic biopsy. One of the golden rules of medicine is this: DON'T LOOK FOR SOMETHING IF YOU'RE NOT GOING TO DO ANYTHING WHEN YOU FIND IT!

How Is a Biopsy Performed?

A biopsy is obtained by inserting a needle into the prostate. This can be accomplished via one of two routes. In a transperineal biopsy, the needle is introduced through the perineum, the area between the scrotum and the anus. A transrectal biopsy is taken through the wall of the rectum. Both methods are equally accurate, so the decision as to which is used is based upon the physician's preference.

Transrectal and transperineal biopsies are both core biopsies, which means the needle actually cuts a cylinder-shaped core from the prostate tissue much as you might core an apple. A long, thin, wire-like insert is placed within the barrel of the needle to close the hole until the physician is ready to collect the biopsy. In the transrectal method, the physician holds the needle against the tip of his index finger and places the needle-and-finger combination into the rectum. The needle is then passed through the rectal wall into the prostate gland until the suspicious area is reached, at which point the insert is removed and the core is taken. The transperineal biopsy is done in a similar manner, except the needle is inserted through the perineum as the physician's finger locates the target area through the rectum. Transrectal and transperineal biopsies both can be performed with or without local anesthesia. But both types are being performed less often since the advent of transrectal ultrasound (TRUS)-guided biopsies.

Proponents of transperineal biopsy argue that their technique carries a lower risk of infection because it does not involve passing a needle through the rectum. The risk of infection historically has been the primary disadvantage of transrectal biopsies, which is why an enema and an antibiotic are given before the procedure is performed. However, recent advances in biopsy technology have made this much less of a consideration. Smaller needles mounted on spring-loaded biopsy guns and ultrasound-guided needle placement have made post-biopsy infections a rare occurrence. If a serious possibility of prostate cancer exists, the most important issue is not the route of biopsy collection, but that the biopsy is obtained.

What Is Fine-Needle Aspiration?

Fine-needle aspiration (FNA) is similar to biopsy, but uses a much finer needle. Rather than cutting a core of tissue from the prostate, the FNA technique applies suction with a syringe as the needle is passed in and out of the gland. The sample obtained is a representative collection of cells, instead of a piece of the organ.

The thinner needle gives FNA a much lower risk of infection than transrectal core biopsy, and the results of the test are usually available within hours. However, FNA has yet to gain wide acceptance in the U.S., because it requires the presence of a pathologist who is specially trained in examining FNA specimens. This is not a problem in most major university medical centers, but it can be in many of the smaller community hospitals. Any advantage gained in decreasing the risk of infection is overshadowed by the risk of obtaining an unreliable diagnosis.

What Is Transrectal Ultrasound?

Today's ultrasound technology is used to evaluate everything from unborn fetuses to heart valves to gallbladders. Its safety and accuracy have made it an indispensible tool in diagnosing and treating many disease processes, including prostate cancer. Ultrasound operates like a radar device. An ultrasound transmitter sends sound waves at a frequency too high for humans to hear. When these waves strike a solid object, they are absorbed or reflected to a certain degree, depending on the consistency of the object. The altered waves echo back to a receiver and a computerized detector converts them into a visual image.

When transrectal ultrasound (TRUS) was first introduced, it was expected to revolutionize the staging of prostate cancer. Unfortunately, it is little better, if at all, than DRE, and experts have yet to agree on what its routine use will eventually be. One advantage TRUS does have over DRE is that it can reveal if cancer has spread to the seminal vesicles.

At present, TRUS is used most frequently in precisely locating suspicious areas for biopsy. In this capacity, it is superb. It allows direct visualization of the biopsy needle at all times and makes certain that the part of the prostate in which the physician is interested is reached. TRUS is also very useful in measuring the size of the prostate gland and in examining the capsule for any signs of cancer spread.

TRUS does have some role in the early detection of cancer. Many cancers that are not detected by DRE are eventually found by TRUS. Additionally, cancers that are poorly differentiated (high-grade) are more visible on TRUS than well-differentiated (low-grade) tumors. As with DRE, any suspicious area that is found by TRUS should be biopsied.

It is important to think of TRUS and DRE not as two independent diagnostic tests, but as two members of the same team, each with its strengths and weaknesses. In fact, when a third team member, prostate-specific antigen (PSA), is added to the diagnostic workup, the accuracies of the other two are enhanced tremendously. An abnormal DRE or TRUS in the setting of a normal PSA means the suspicious area is most likely not cancerous. On the other hand, an elevated PSA with an abnormal TRUS or DRE suggests a high likelihood that cancer will be found on biopsy. Therefore, DRE, TRUS, and PSA should always be thought of as a diagnostic triad rather than three individual tests. A definite abnormality on any should be followed by a biopsy.

My Biopsy Shows Cancer. Now What?

Once a diagnosis of cancer has been made, it is essential to know the degree of advancement or stage of the tumor before a treatment modality can be chosen. Carcinoma localized to the prostate (stage A or B) can potentially be cured with surgery or radiation therapy, whereas cancer that has left the gland and invaded other structures (stage C or D) cannot. The goal of staging, therefore, is to evaluate lymph nodes and organs outside the prostate for the presence of cancer. Many different tests and procedures are used for this purpose.

Blood tests are usually done early in the staging process, because they are quick, easy, and can provide valuable information. The PSA is obviously the most important blood test in evaluating prostate cancer, especially in the period after treatment. Abnormal liver function tests (LFTs), such as bilirubin and the transaminases, can suggest metastases to that organ. A decreased red blood cell count might signify bone marrow involvement or the anemia that often accompanies a chronic disease. Kidney function tests, such as creatinine and blood urea nitrogen (BUN) that are elevated in the setting of prostate cancer, raise the possibility of obstruction of the ureter, the tube that carries urine from the kidney to the bladder. It is important to remember that none of these tests are diagnostic in and of themselves. They must all be interpreted in the context of other test results.

Cystoscopy was once an essential part of prostate cancer staging, but is used less frequently today. In this procedure, a special telescope is inserted into the urethra through the opening at the end of the penis and advanced into the bladder. This allows the urologist to check for extension of the tumor into the bladder and urethra. Anesthesia beyond numbing of the urethra and mild sedation is rarely necessary for this procedure. Cystoscopy can usually be performed at the same time as the biopsy and TRUS.

Cystoscopy, while an excellent means of evaluating the bladder and urethra, is unable to visualize the ureters. If obstruction of a ureter by a metastasis is suspected (on the basis of an elevated BUN and creatinine, for example), the best test to confirm it is intravenous pyelography (IVP). This is a radiologic study in which dye is injected through an intravenous catheter and x-rays are taken as the dye passes through the kidneys and ureters.

As we have learned, the most common site for distant prostate cancer metastases is bone. The best test for ruling out bony metastases is bone scintigraphy or bone scan. In this radiologic study, radioactive technetium-99 is injected into the body, where it attaches to areas of bone that have a high rate of buildup and degradation. A picture of the body then is taken and areas where large amounts of technetium have accumulated will "light up."

PSA is a good predictor of when a bone scan is likely to show metastases, so this study should be performed whenever prostate cancer is confirmed and the blood PSA level is markedly elevated. A bone scan should also be done if you have been diagnosed with prostate cancer and you experience bone pain. Bone scans are not very specific for metastases, however. Any disease process that causes a high bone turnover rate, such as arthritis, Paget's disease, or a healing fracture, will yield a positive bone scan.

What Is a Pelvic Lymph Node Dissection?

Pelvic lymph node dissection (PLND), the surgical removal and pathologic examination of pelvic lymph nodes, is arguably the most important staging procedure of all and is the last step taken before forging ahead with radiation therapy or radical prostatectomy. You must fulfill two criteria before you can be considered a candidate for PLND: first, all tests preceding the PLND must indicate that your cancer is localized to the prostate (stage A, B, or very early C); and second, you must be willing and medically fit to undergo radiation therapy or radical surgery if the lymph nodes are found to be free of cancer. You and your doctor should also decide before the PLND which treatment modality you will pursue if the lymph nodes are negative.

PLND is essential because invasion of the lymph nodes by cancer cells greatly affects whether or not treatment will be successful. Most men who have a negative staging workup until PLND reveals positive lymph nodes end up having metastases in other organs a few years later. The number of positive lymph nodes does make a difference, however. One positive node is better than two, and microscopic tumor infiltration is better than visible involvement. As discussed in the previous chapter, the grade also matters; a high-grade tumor is more likely to metastasize to the lymph nodes than a low-grade.

Traditional PLNDs are done under general anesthesia through an incision below the belly button and above the pubic area. The surgeon makes his way into the pelvis without actually entering the abdominal cavity (an extraperitoneal approach), a technique that reduces the risk of infection and internal scar tissue formation. Once he reaches the pelvis, the surgeon removes a representative sample of lymph nodes from both sides. It is important to leave some lymph nodes behind in order to avoid postoperative complications like swelling of the legs; removing all of the pelvic lymph nodes does not improve chances for cure. The entire operation takes about 90 minutes to complete and requires about a week's hospitalization afterward.

PLND is a major operation and thus carries certain risks. Wound complications, like infection or the accumulation of lymphatic fluid under the skin, can occur. The possibility of nerve or blood vessel injury exists as well. That most men undergoing PLND for prostate cancer are in their sixties or older also increases the risk of this procedure. Having to do a PLND is particularly unfortunate if radiation therapy is being chosen, because it erases this treatment option's primary advantage of not requiring surgery.

For these reasons laparoscopic PLND was developed. This procedure is performed by inserting a special telescope and other surgical instruments through several small stab wounds in the abdomen. It is equally as effective as the traditional PLND and involves a much shorter hospital stay (24–36 hours) and a much quicker return to normal activity. In addition, more and more surgeons are gaining experience performing laparoscopy extraperitoneally, thus avoiding the complications that arise when the abdominal cavity is entered.

If you choose radiation therapy as your treatment, the PLND will obviously have to be done as a separate procedure. If you choose surgery, however, PLND can be done at the same time. This is called one-step surgery and its main advantage is that it avoids a second operation. In this treatment strategy, the surgeon prepares himself and the operating room as if radical prostatectomy were to take place. The PLND is done first and a specimen is sent to the pathology laboratory for a frozen section, so the pathologist can examine the lymph nodes for cancer invasion and give an opinion within minutes. If the lymph nodes are positive, the operation is ended and alternate therapies (i.e., hormonal) are discussed; if the nodes are negative, the prostatectomy proceeds. The pathologist then prepares a permanent section from the lymph nodes, which is more accurate than the frozen section, but requires several days to complete.

The problem with one-step surgery is that the permanent section frequently disagrees with the frozen. If surgery is done on the basis of a negative frozen section and the permanent section later shows lymph node metastases, then an unnecessary operation has been performed. Therefore, you may want to consider two-step surgery. As with radiation therapy, two-step surgery involves performing PLND as a separate procedure. The more reliable permanent section results can be used to determine whether prostatectomy is feasible. Laparoscopic PLND has made two-step surgery a much safer option than it used to be.

Can CT Scans and MRIs Be Used for Staging?

A CT (computerized tomography) scan is a sophisticated ring-shaped x-ray machine that takes computerized "slices" of the body and converts them into photographic images. It has been used quite a bit not only for examining the prostate itself, but in assisting lymph node biopsies in cases of diagnosed prostate cancer. The problem with CT scans in assessing lymph nodes is that the nodes must *look* visibly abnormal in order to arouse suspicion. This means lymph nodes with microscopic metastases will slip through the cracks. For this reason many experts consider the CT's role in prostate cancer staging to be limited.

MRI (magnetic resonance imaging) has similar disadvantages. This technique uses a giant tunnel-shaped magnet to obtain strikingly detailed pictures of internal organs and structures. Like the CT scan, however, it cannot detect microscopic invasion. In addition, the traditional whole-body MRI makes "slices" that are too thick for close examination of a tiny organ like the prostate. The study also takes a long time to complete, the machine makes loud noises, and its tunnel causes many patients to feel claustrophobic. Current research into an MRI coil placed in the rectum may eventually solve these problems.

Are There Any Other Areas of Staging Research?

Yes. A great deal of interest currently is focused on the DNA content of tumor cells. DNA is deoxyribonucleic acid, a highly complex molecule that is the genetic code determining all of our inherited traits. Everything from the color of our eyes to the shape of our earlobes to our tendency to contract genetic diseases is determined by DNA. DNA is present within every cell of the body in the form of 23 pairs of chromosomes. We each inherit a haploid number (23) of chromosomes from our mother and a haploid number (23) from our father in order to form a complete diploid set (46) of chromosomes.

Scientists have discovered that cancer cells often contain an abnormal or aneuploid, number of chromosomes and that the degree of aneuploidy is related to the aggressiveness and metastatic potential of a tumor. Experts think this is because aneuploid cells can mutate their genetic code at a high rate that allows them to progress rapidly. Aneuploidy consistently has been shown to correlate with the stage, grade, and PSA level of prostate cancer. Aneuploid tumors are more likely to have a high Gleason score, and thus follow a more malignant course than diploid tumors.

Ploidy (whether a tumor is diploid or aneuploid) is determined by a process called DNA flow cytometry, which uses an argon laser to examine the chromosomes of cancer cells. Flow cytometry was developed to address the need for a more objective and predictable measure of malignant potential than the Gleason score. The technology shows promise, but is still experimental.

How Do I Tie All This Together?

The staging of prostate cancer is fraught with difficulties. Many tests, such as DRE and TRUS, are highly subjective, and it is not unusual for two doctors to disagree in inter-

---

Table 3.1
Partial List of Staging Procedures

1. Digital Rectal Examination (DRE)
2. Transrectal Ultrasound (TRUS)
3. Prostate-Specific Antigen (PSA)
4. Biopsy
   a. Core
   b. Fine-Needle Aspiration (FNA)
5. Blood Tests
   a. Complete Blood Count (CBC)
   b. Liver Function Tests (LFTs)
   c. Blood Urea Nitrogen (BUN) & Creatinine
6. Cystoscopy
7. Pelvic Lymph Node Dissection (PLND)
   a. Open PLND
   b. Laparoscopic PLND
8. Bone Scan
9. Intravenous Pyelography (IVP)
10. Magnetic Resonance Imaging (MRI)
11. Computerized Tomography (CT scan)
12. DNA Flow Cytometry

preting the same tumor. Another problem is that benign prostatic hyperplasia (BPH) can give off many of the same signals as cancer and physicians often initiate extensive workups only to find out there was a false alarm. In fact, staging prior to surgery frequently is little more than an educated guess, because of the frequent occurrence of microscopic metastases. The ability of staging to predict which cases of apparently localized cancer are destined to reappear after treatment is less than adequate.

The most important thing to remember is that each case of prostate cancer is unique. There is no single step-by-step algorithm that can be followed in staging this disease. The tests you and your doctor select (Table 3.1) will depend not only on the results of other tests, but also on the treatment plan you devise. If you decide aggressive treatment is right for you, make every effort to rule out metastases beforehand.

Chapter 4

What Is Prostate-Specific Antigen?

That you purchased this book means you probably have heard of prostate-specific antigen (PSA). PSA undoubtedly is the most controversial aspect of the very controversial subject of prostate cancer diagnosis and treatment. In the few short years since PSA first became widely used, countless articles have appeared in the lay and professional press heralding it as a revolutionary find. Because of all this attention PSA merits its own chapter.

The protein that would eventually be called PSA was discovered in 1971 in samples of semen and was named *gamma-seminoprotein*, found to play a role in liquifying semen at ejaculation. In 1979, the substance was isolated in the laboratory and was noted to be specific to the prostate—it was produced *only* by the prostate and *nowhere* else. The significance of this discovery cannot be overstated. Before discovery of PSA, the most effective tool for detection of prostate cancer was acid phosphatase, which, as we learned in chapter 1, is only one of the many components of prostatic fluid. The problem with using acid phosphatase in this capacity is that it also appears in other tissues, namely blood cells and bone. Therefore, an elevation in someone's acid phosphatase level could signify anything from osteoporosis to multiple myeloma to hemolytic anemia. But, thanks to PSA, medical science has its first and only organ-specific cancer marker; no such indicator is available for any other organ! In 1980, PSA was first detected in the blood and its concentration there was found to fluctuate in the setting of various prostate diseases, thus leading the way to the PSA blood tests we now use. The PSA test has all but made the (prostatic) acid phosphatase test obsolete and most experts have stopped it.

How Is PSA Measured?

Two PSA assay devices are currently being used in the U.S., the Tandem®-R by Hybritech® and the IMx® by Abbott®. Other assays exist and are either used in other countries or have FDA applications pending at this writing. All of the tests utilize antibodies specifically designed to bind to PSA; attached to each antibody molecule is a tiny radioactive label. The more PSA that is present in the blood, the more radioactive-labeled antibody that will bind to it, and the higher the reading will be.

A man with a normal prostate should have almost no PSA in his blood. It is only after some process has disrupted the architecture of the gland that the protein is able to infiltrate the prostatic tissue and gain access to the blood circulation. Both benign prostatic hyperplasia (BPH) and carcinoma of the prostate can do this and cause an elevated blood PSA level; that is what makes the test so valuable. Unfortunately, many other things can also lead to an increased PSA value. Prostate infections, dead prostatic tissue, urinary retention, and bladder catheterization are a few of the other noncancerous causes of PSA elevation. Certain procedures your doctor performs, such as cystoscopy, transrectal ultrasound (TRUS), prostatic biopsy, transurethral resection (TURP), and to a lesser degree, digital rectal examination (DRE), also can release PSA into the blood. For this reason, it is best to draw blood for a PSA test before or wait until two or three weeks after any such manipulations are done; 48 hours is sufficient following a DRE.

PSA blood levels are measured in nanograms (billionths of a gram!) per milliliter (about ⅟₃₀ of a fluid ounce). A level below 4 ng/ml is considered normal and reflects a low risk for prostate cancer; the risk is not zero, however, as cancers do occur in the setting of "normal" PSA concentrations. A PSA reading greater than 10 ng/ml clearly represents a high risk for carcinoma and warrants a biopsy. The intermediate range between 4.1 and 10 ng/ml has led to much of the controversy surrounding PSA, because this is where most of the overlap between BPH and cancer occurs. More than a few experts recommend biopsy for any PSA value greater than 4 ng/ml, but many others are currently trying to modify use of PSA levels in an attempt to separate cancers from BPHs.

Considerable research is being directed at changing the assays themselves. Monitoring PSA levels after treatment is the single best use of this test. A rising PSA after an initial decline following radiation therapy or surgery is a telltale sign of residual cancer. Therefore, the sooner this turnaround can be detected, the sooner additional therapy can be instituted. New ultrasensitive assays, which can measure PSA levels that are undetectable by present methods, are currently being investigated.

Will My BPH Medicine Affect My PSA Level?

If you're taking Proscar® (finasteride), yes. This is a new medication that reduces the size of the prostate gland and, consequently, the PSA level. If you have been taking Proscar® for 12 months or more, your PSA will be half what it would be without the drug. Therefore, your doctor still can follow your PSA readings simply by multiplying the result by two. This only works if you have been taking your medicine as directed for 12 months or more. If you have skipped or combined doses, the PSA will be unreliable.

Does the PSA Level Rise as Cancer Grows?

Not only does the PSA rise with cancer growth, but the degree of PSA increase is directly proportional to the change in the size of the tumor. For each gram (about ⅟₃₀ of an ounce) of new cancer tissue, the PSA can be expected to rise by 3.5 ng/ml. This applies to all of the cancerous tissue that is present, including that which has penetrated the capsule or metastasized to other organs. A similar, but more gradual, relationship exists between the PSA level and BPH; for each gram of new BPH tissue, the PSA increases by 0.3 ng/ml.

Unfortunately, while the PSA concentration is an excellent means of estimating changes in tumor size, it cannot accurately predict tumor stage on an individual basis. In other words, your doctor cannot look at your PSA value and tell whether or not your cancer has spread beyond the prostate. Any given PSA level can be associated with a wide range of cancer stages in different people. For example, Martin W. had a PSA of 15 ng/ml and a tumor that was confined to the prostate, whereas Jonathan F. had the same PSA with metastatic disease.

While PSA measurements cannot stage cancers on a person-by-person basis, they can be used to gauge the likelihood of cancer spread. For example, a tumor with a PSA of 30 ng/ml is more likely to have metastasized than one with a PSA of 12 ng/ml, especially if the Gleason score shows an aggressive cell type. In fact, the PSA level is probably the best way to predict if your bone scan will end up showing metastases to the bone. Most experts agree that if you have a newly diagnosed cancer with no symptoms and a PSA less than 10 ng/ml, or even less than 20 ng/ml, it is not necessary to perform a bone scan.

Can PSA Be Used to Screen People for Cancer?

Screening is the testing of people in the general population who have no symptoms in order to identify those who are more likely to have a given disease. Many different screening tests exist for many different diseases. Guaiac cards for detecting blood in the stool are used to screen for colon cancer. Blood pressure booths are set up in shopping malls to screen people for hypertension. These are effective screening tests, because they are simple, inexpensive, and they can reduce the number of deaths or serious complications that would occur in the absence of screening. The cost to society of a good screening test is far less than the cost of not doing the test.

As of 1995, the Food and Drug Administration (FDA) has approved the use of PSA only in monitoring prostate cancer after treatment, not as a screening test. Even so, most doctors use PSA testing for screening purposes anyway, which is perfectly legal. A physician is allowed to use a test or medication in a nonapproved manner if he believes it is in his patient's best interest; this is called clinical judgment. Many experts support PSA as a screening modality, because they believe that using a test that has the potential to detect cancer at an early stage when treatment is most likely to be successful is better than allowing tumors to progress. It is hard to argue with this logic! In fact, the American Cancer Society (ACS) and the American Urological Association (AUA) currently recommend annual PSA testing for all men over 50 (40 for black men and men with a significant family history), so it is clear that screening is widely endorsed, even in the absence of FDA approval.

There are those who oppose screening for prostate cancer with PSA testing, and their arguments are quite convincing. For a screening test to be worthwhile, it must be shown to improve survival statistics, meaning it must reduce the number of people who die specifically from the disease itself. The problem with PSA testing is that, while it can detect tumors at a less-advanced stage, it has not been shown to decrease prostate cancer mortality. In other words, the average life expectancy of a man with prostate cancer today has changed little since the days before the PSA assay became widely used. This is mainly because most prostate tumors grow very slowly and most men who have prostate cancer are in the latter part of their lifespan anyway. It does not make sense to search for a small tumor that will take 10 years to kill the man carrying it if that man is likely to die from other causes in 8 years! Statistics show that MORE MEN DIE *WITH* PROSTATE CANCER THAN *FROM* PROSTATE CANCER! Mortality figures will improve only when tests can identify the minority of men who have rapidly growing tumors and will therefore be saved by early detection of their disease.

Opponents of PSA screening also state that the test is not specific or sensitive enough to be used for this purpose. Specificity reflects a test's ability to detect the disease of interest and ignore other diseases. A very specific test will have few false positives, meaning that few people without the disease will have a positive test result. Sensitivity refers to a test's success in picking out people with the disease from a crowd. A sensitive test will have few false negatives, which are people who have the disease, but get a negative test result. The PSA test is considered insensitive, because many men with small cancers have normal PSA readings. The new ultrasensitive assays may improve this eventually. The test is very specific for prostate tissue, because PSA is not produced by any other organ. Unfortunately, while PSA is specific for the prostate, it is not specific for prostate *cancer*.

The specificity of PSA testing for prostate cancer is compromised by the fact that most men with cancer also have a certain degree of benign enlargement (BPH), which increases the PSA level and is far more common than cancer. PSA elevations are therefore more likely to be caused by BPH than cancer, especially in the 4.1 to 10 ng/ml range. When cancer is present, it is usually of a heterogeneous nature, with several different cell groups of varying degrees of aggressiveness. Cancers with a high Gleason score tend to be larger and more disruptive of the prostatic architecture, thus leading to a higher PSA value, than less aggressive tumors, but the production of PSA per cell is actually *lower* in high-grade cells. This further affects the specificity of PSA testing.

What Can Be Done to Improve Sensitivity and Specificity?

Five different PSA modifications (Table 4.1) are currently being investigated to improve the test's sensitivity and specificity for prostate cancer: PSA density, PSA cancer

---

Table 4.1
Proposed Modifications of PSA Testing to
Enhance Sensitivity and Specificity

---

1. PSA Density (PSAD)
2. PSA Cancer Density (PSACD)
3. Age-Specific Reference Ranges
4. PSA Velocity (DPSA)
5. PSA-ACT Complexes

---

density, PSA velocity, age-specific reference ranges, and PSA-ACT complexes.

PSA density (PSAD) is merely the PSA blood level divided by the volume of the prostate gland, as measured by transrectal ultrasound (TRUS), because usually there is a greater total volume of tissue producing PSA in the presence of cancer than in BPH. Factoring in prostatic volume helps separate PSA elevations from cancer from those caused by BPH. PSAD is particularly useful in the 4.1 to 10 ng/ml range, where most cancer-BPH overlap occurs. Some studies have shown that if PSAD is greater than 0.15, chances are better than 80 percent that the PSA is elevated because of cancer. Opponents of PSAD tests believe it leaves too much overlap between BPH and cancer to justify the high cost of TRUS.

TRUS-measured prostate volume is also needed to calculate PSA cancer density (PSACD)—PSA level multiplied by the volume of the tumor, then divided by the volume of the prostate gland. PSACD cannot be used to detect early cancer, because the cancer has to be identified before its volume can be measured. Even so, it is superior to PSAD in predicting which tumors will eventually show themselves

Table 4.2
Age-Specific Reference Ranges for PSA Level

Age Range	Upper Limit of Normal (ng/ml)
40–49	2.5
50–59	3.5
60–69	4.5
70–79	6.5

to have higher Gleason scores and to have spread to other organs, invaluable in planning further tests and treatment. PSACD's primary disadvantage: the present methods for measuring cancer volume are still inadequate. Rectal MRI coils may do better.

As a man ages, he can expect an increase in his PSA level whether or not he has BPH or cancer, because the prostate gland has a natural tendency to become larger and "leakier" with age. While it may be reasonable to expect a 35-year-old man to have a PSA value below 4 ng/ml, it may not be reasonable to expect that in a 75 year old. Therefore many researchers are proposing to adopt age-specific reference ranges (Table 4.2). Lowering the upper limit of normal in younger men increases the sensitivity of PSA testing, because it will then detect more tumors in the age group that benefits most from aggressive treatment. Raising the limit for older men improves specificity, because fewer men end up having unnecessary biopsies and other procedures. Because age-specific reference ranges accomplish everything PSAD does and more, they show considerable promise for eventually gaining wide acceptance.

Another PSA modification takes into account that PSA rises much quicker in a cancer setting than when BPH is present. The PSA velocity (ΔPSA) measures the rate of change in PSA value over a given time; at least two separate values must be obtained in order to measure it. ΔPSA may prove to be the most practical use of the PSA assay. ΔPSAs greater than 0.75 ng/ml per year have a specificity for cancer that exceeds 90 percent, which may be especially valuable when assessing men with mildly elevated PSA levels and normal DREs and TRUSs.

When PSA escapes from the prostate and enters the bloodstream, it rarely circulates as a free, independent molecule. Instead, it usually binds to another molecule to form a complex. The two chemicals PSA forms complexes with most frequently are alpha-2-macroglobulin (α2M) and alpha-1-antichymotrypsin (ACT). ACT is manufactured primarily in the liver, but small amounts also are made in the prostate. Researchers are not sure about the significance of PSA-α2M complexes, but the importance of PSA-ACT complexes is clear. The percentage of PSA-ACT complexes in people with prostate cancer is much higher than in BPH cases. Conversely, the proportion of free PSA is higher in BPH than cancer. Therefore, utilizing the ratio of PSA-ACT complexes to the total PSA concentration can greatly enhance the specificity of PSA testing for cancer. As with the other modifications, using PSA complexes to diagnose prostate cancer is still experimental.

If My Cancer Is Treated, Will My PSA Level Go Down?

Provided the treatment is successful, yes. In fact, monitoring prostate cancer after treatment is the single best and only FDA-approved use of the PSA test. Thanks to PSA, doctors and patients no longer have to wait for symptoms to develop before they know whether treatment was effective. PSA changes can precede symptoms by months or even years, so that additional therapy can begin sooner. The basic rule of prostate cancer treatment: IF THE PSA IS RISING, THE TUMOR IS GROWING. An important corollary: if the PSA is not rising, the tumor still could be growing, which can happen in 1 out of 5 cases.

When a radical prostatectomy is performed, the surgeon's goal is to remove *all* prostatic tissue from the patient's body. Since PSA is produced only in the prostate, if a prostatectomy is successful, that should cause PSA to disappear from the blood. Normally it takes two to three weeks for PSA to become undetectable, but if PSA is still detected in the blood after a radical prostatectomy, residual cancer is still present, so the possibility of instituting adjuvant therapy (i.e., radiation) probably should be raised. Adjuvant therapy is discussed in greater detail in chapter 5.

Additional therapy is usually not feasible until at least three months after such a major operation, so many physicians wait until then to measure postoperative PSA level. Even if the PSA is undetectable three months after surgery, your doctor will still want to monitor your levels for a while, because some cancer recurrences take years to appear. The longer it takes, the better your prognosis. PSA levels measured before surgery are good predictors of recurrence. Higher preoperative PSAs can mean a greater risk of lymph node metastasis and recurrence.

Pretreatment PSA concentration is even more important to monitor radiation therapy; the higher the level, the poorer the outcome is likely to be. Monitoring PSA after radiation is a little trickier, because the prostate is not removed, so it is still producing PSA. Within 6 months after radiation, the PSA should fall to normal but detectable levels. Most successful treatments result in normalization by 3 months, but some PSA levels continue to fall for as long as 12 months. A PSA reading exceeding 4 ng/ml at 6 months indicates treatment failure. Therapy can also be considered to have failed if the PSA is above 10 ng/ml at 3 months. An increase in PSA any time after treatment is indicative of residual tumor, so adjuvant therapy (i.e., hormonal) should be considered.

Men who undergo hormonal therapy generally have tumors more advanced than those treatable by surgery or radiation, so a less-dramatic PSA change is usually expected. As with the other treatment modalities, the goal is to reach the range of normal and the sooner the better. A decline in the PSA concentration within 3 months to 4 ng/ml that is maintained for at least 6 months is the best predictor of a long-term response to therapy. Even if the PSA remains normal, however, the possibility of a growing tumor always exists. As with prostatectomy and radiation, if the PSA rises after hormonal therapy, the tumor is recurring. New ultrasensitive PSA assays may soon aid early detection of prostate cancer recurrences.

When Should I Have My PSA Checked?

The PSA assay is fairly new, so it is not surprising that experts disagree on its ideal application. Clearly, it is valuable for monitoring prostate cancer after treatment. It will probably be of equal value in cancer screening, but it may take 10 to 15 years before current research studies can determine whether PSA testing reduces mortality. PSA *is* organ-specific and, unlike DRE and TRUS, is entirely objective, so its role in diagnosing and treating prostate disease will be significant, regardless of the final verdict.

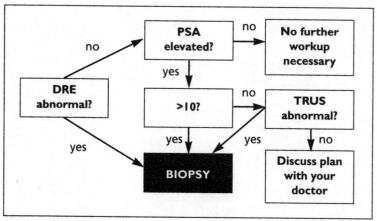

Figure 4.1: Algorithm for combining PSA, DRE, and TRUS results to diagnose prostate cancer.

For now, the American Cancer Society and the American Urological Association recommend that every man beginning at age 50 have his PSA tested annually. Black men and men with a significant family history should begin checking PSA levels at 40. Men with a life expectancy of less than 10 years are unlikely to benefit from aggressive treatment and need not bother to have their PSAs checked. The PSA should only be interpreted in the context of other test results, and the value of DRE, TRUS, and biopsy should not be underestimated. Figure 4.1 illustrates one way of tying these tests together, but this is only one of many possible combinations.

What Types of Prostate Surgery Are There?

Prostate operations have been around for decades, but most men with prostate cancer have been reluctant to select them as their choice of treatment. Most traditional prostate surgical procedures involved substantial blood loss, a 50 percent chance of urinary incontinence (loss of bladder control), and a near-100 percent chance of impotence (loss of erections), so it's no wonder so many men considered the treatment worse than the disease. Ten years ago, only 1 man in 10 with prostate cancer was treated surgically. Today, that figure is 1 in 4. Obviously, some drastic changes in prostate surgery have occurred during this period for so many more men to embrace such a previously unpopular treatment.

One major change is that methods of early cancer detection like PSA and ultrasound have become much more prevalent, so more men can have their cancers diagnosed sooner (stage A or B), when surgery can cure the disease, and when the men are younger, reducing surgical complication risks. Another factor making surgery more popular is that most of the serious complications that were troublesome in the past have been solved to a great extent. A team of prominent urologists took a meticulous look at the anatomy of the prostate and the structures surrounding it, something that had not been done. They were able to find the source of the bleeding that was giving surgeons so much trouble: the dorsal vein. Today, the dorsal vein can be identified and tied off early in the operation, before it can bleed at all. These same anatomic studies yielded an even greater discovery that would lead to development of the nerve-sparing radical prostatectomy and a real revolution in prostate cancer treatment.

What Is the Nerve-Sparing Radical Prostatectomy?

Men who underwent most older prostate operations typically became impotent. Because surgeons at that time were unfamiliar with the nerves responsible for erection, the nerve supplying the erection-causing part of the penis, the corpus cavernosum, was usually cut inadvertently. Even if they had known what to look for, they would have had a hard time seeing past all the bleeding from the dorsal vein. The same anatomic studies that identified the dorsal vein led to identification of the erection-causing nerve.

The pelvic plexus is a twisted intersection of multiple nerve fibers located on the side wall of the rectum. The pelvic plexus sends nerve branches to many organs within the pelvis, including a branch that goes to the corpus cavernosum of the penis. This nerve branch and the blood vessels that run beside it are packaged together as a neurovascular bundle. The primary advantage of the nerve-sparing radical prostatectomy, and the reason most men who have it are able to retain their ability to have erections, is that this neurovascular bundle is left intact.

However, the most important goal of the nerve-sparing radical prostatectomy or any other cancer operation is to remove *all* of the tumor. The second most important goal is to maintain bladder function; few men care about attaining an erection when they can't hold their urine. This puts preserving sexual function third on the list, and sometimes at least one of the two neurovascular bundles (usually the one on the side of the tumor) has to be cut in order to remove all of the cancer. This doesn't happen very often, but when it does it usually doesn't matter, because one neurovascular bundle is all most men need to be able to achieve erection.

What Type of Incision Does the Operation Require?

Today, the nerve-sparing radical prostatectomy usually is done through a retropubic (behind the pubic bone) approach. A vertical incision is made between the belly button and the pubic area. As discussed in chapter 3, a pelvic lymph node dissection can also be performed through this incision. The lymph nodes are sent to the pathology lab for a frozen section and if positive for cancer, the disease is too far advanced for surgery to help, so the incision is closed. If the nodes come back negative, the operation proceeds.

Radical prostatectomy involves removing the entire prostate gland and seminal vesicles. The operation also removes a man's ability to sire children, because the two vasa deferens are cut and tied as in a vasectomy. The last part of the procedure involves reconstructing the bladder and reattaching it to the urethra. All this is done while the surgeon pays careful attention to the neurovascular bundles and the dorsal vein. Tremendous technical skill is required to perform this procedure.

What Can I Expect After the Operation?

After a nerve-sparing radical retropubic prostatectomy, you can expect to remain in the hospital about a week. You will probably notice a few tubes coming out of your body when you awaken after surgery. A couple of them will be suction drains, which stay in place for several days to remove blood and fluid from the area where your prostate used to be. A Foley catheter will be in your urethra to drain urine from your bladder into a plastic bag. Most likely, you will leave the hospital with the Foley catheter still in place. Your doctor will remove it in his office about two weeks after the operation, which is usually how long it takes the reconstructed bladder to heal.

The nerve-sparing procedure promises retained potency in most men, but it usually returns slowly. Most men will achieve erections within 3 to 6 months after surgery, but some take as long as 18 months. Unfortunately, 30 percent or so, like Richard M., will remain impotent. Whether you will become impotent from the surgery depends greatly upon your age and the stage of your tumor. From 80–90 percent of men under 50 remain potent after nerve-sparing prostatectomy, unlike only 15–25 percent of men in their 70s. In avoiding impotence, stage A1 is better than A2 is better than B1 is better than B2

Like potency, urinary continence also returns slowly after surgery, sometimes taking 6 months or longer. The odds of regaining complete continence after radical prostatectomy are 95 percent, however, so try your best to remain patient while your urinary control returns. Most of the 5 percent of men who do not regain full urinary control have stress incontinence, which means they can hold their urine most of the time and are incontinent only when there is increased pressure on the bladder (i.e., when sneezing, coughing, or lifting). Age is also an important factor in predicting incontinence after surgery. Curiously, potency and continence do not appear to be related. One has nothing to do with the other.

Several other potential complications can develop after nerve-sparing radical prostatectomy, but, fortunately, they are rare. Lying in bed after the operation increases the likelihood of blood clots forming in the legs (deep venous thrombosis). Not only can these blood clots cause problems in their own right, like leg swelling and inflammation (thrombophlebitis), they can also break off and float upstream until becoming trapped in the lungs. Called pulmonary embolism, this is a potentially fatal complication. Therefore, your doctor will probably advise you to get out of bed and move around soon after the procedure.

Wound infections are possible complications with any operation, and radical prostatectomy is no exception. Collections of lymphatic fluid (lymphocele) at the site of the pelvic lymph node dissection can occur. A narrowing of the bladder's attachment to the urethra may also develop, but your urologist can fix that by passing a dilator through the urethra. Don't be alarmed by this list of complications. Most are uncommon, mentioned only so you'll have complete information.

How Do I Correct Incontinence or Impotence?

There are many ways to deal with urinary incontinence. The method you select will depend largely on your personal preference. Herb K. wears an absorbent undergarment. Philip J. uses a condom-like Texas catheter that drains into a bag. Surgical procedures can correct most problems. A newer treatment for incontinence involves injecting collagen around the urethra to increase its bulk and, consequently, its ability to contain leakage. Talk to your urologist.

Impotence after nerve-sparing radical prostatectomy may actually be more prevalent than you might have read, because too little consideration is given to the *quality* of erections in men who are allegedly potent. Stephen F., for example, could achieve a partial erection after his surgery, but it was not rigid enough for him to resume normal sexual activity. That made him very upset, understandably. He was resigned to the condition, largely because he was too embarassed to talk to his doctor. Not until his wife convinced him help was available did he actually do something.

Do not fall into this trap. If you are dissatisfied with any aspect of your sexual function after surgery (or any other treatment) for prostate cancer, you must let your feelings be known. Many techniques are available today for treating impotence or improving partial erections. Sexual counseling and sensate focus exercises help many people. Urologists have many tools available too, including vacuum erection devices, intracavernous injections, and penile prostheses. Talk to your family and friends and let them know what is on your mind, then talk to your doctor, so you can get an appropriate referral to fix your problem. The best time to begin talking to your doctor about how a treatment will affect your sex life is *before* treatment begins, when postoperative considerations can be incorporated into your care plan.

Are There Other Surgical Approaches Besides Retropubic?

The most popular approach for radical prostatectomy before blood loss was improved in the retropubic operation was the perineal. It is performed through a semicircular incision that surrounds the anus. The primary advantages of perineal prostatectomy over retropubic are that it allows an easier attachment of the bladder to the urethra and it is easier to perform on obese men. Historically, it has involved a much lower blood loss than retropubic prostatectomy, but improvements in the latter have made that less of an issue. The primary *disadvantage* of the perineal operation is that pelvic lymph node dissection requires a separate incision. Laparoscopic lymph node dissections have reduced this effect.

A third surgical approach, rarely used today, is the transcoccygeal approach, which involves an incision between the buttocks and the removal of the tailbone to reach the prostate. As in the perineal approach, the transcoccygeal's primary advantage is easier bladder-urethra attachment; the main disadvantage is also a separate incision for pelvic lymph node dissection.

The important thing to remember about retropubic, perineal, and transcoccygeal approaches to radical prostatectomy is that they are equally effective in treating prostate cancer and all can be done using a nerve-sparing technique. Therefore, the choice among the three should depend solely on the expertise of your urologist.

How Do I Decide If Surgery Is Right for Me?

The debate over which treatment method, if any, is best for treating prostate cancer is one of the most passionate in medical science. The war over surgery vs. radiation vs. hormones vs. watching-and-waiting has been raging for years and shows no signs of slowing. Despite this controversy, no treatment modality has been proved clearly superior to the rest. How you choose to treat your prostate cancer will depend more on what is available in your area and to whom you speak than almost anything else. If you talk to a radiation oncologist or if your hospital has a good radiation oncology department, you are likelier to pursue radiation therapy. But if you have access to a highly experienced urologist, surgery will probably be your choice. There is nothing wrong with this strategy. There is considerable overlap between these territories and they are almost equally effective.

A man's likelihood of dying from prostate cancer appears to be the same with or without treatment, prompting some people to ask whether treatment is necessary at all. We will address this question in chapter 8. This chapter and the two following it will attempt an unbiased assessment of surgery, radiation therapy, and hormonal therapy. Only you, with the help of your doctor, can make a therapy choice. That decision should be an informed one, so these chapters will try to provide as much relevant information as possible from all sides.

Radical prostatectomy is best for men whose cancer is confined to the prostate (stage A or B) and who have at least 10 to 15 years of life expectancy. Within this group, everyone can pursue nerve-sparing techniques except those with stage B2 cancer (inside prostate, both sides). Many stage B2 tumors end up actually as stage C (through capsule) when they are removed and examined in the pathology lab, especially if the cancer cells have a high Gleason score (very aggressive). Therefore, a radical prostatectomy for stage B2 cancer should include removal of the neurovascular bundles to maximize getting all of the cancer. Gene Q. had stage A2 prostate cancer, but had his neurovascular bundles removed anyway because he was impotent before the surgery. His urologist advised him that would allow Gene the best chances for getting all of the tumor.

Few responsible physicians would argue against selecting radiation therapy for stage C cancer, but some believe radiation therapy is best for stage B2 cancer too, especially if it is approaching stage C. That was the case with Bernard D., whose multiple medical problems made him a poor surgical risk. Michael Y., on the other hand, was young and healthy and his doctors thought treating his stage B2 disease with radiation probably was an unnecessarily cautious plan. A lot depends on your individual situation and the philosophy of your physicians. As soon as you are diagnosed with cancer, you should have a long discussion with your doctor to evaluate various treatments, to decide on a treatment modality, and to formulate a contingency plan if something unforeseen should arise.

What If Surgery Doesn't Get All of the Cancer?

When the pathologist receives a cancerous prostate that has been surgically removed, he cuts it into multiple thin slices and examines each one under the microscope. Then he checks the perimeter of the prostate on all sides for signs of cancer. If he finds no evidence of cancer at the outermost aspects of the gland, he can say the margins are negative and all of the cancer is contained within the prostate and was removed. That is the objective of a radical prostatectomy—to remove *all* of the cancer.

Unfortunately, as many as a third of all men who undergo radical prostatectomy have margins that are positive for cancer, which means their surgery failed to remove all the cancer. This usually happens because a doctor's ability to stage cancer before surgery, as we have learned, is mediocre at best. Many tumors initially thought to be stage B (confined to prostate) on the basis of staging procedures end up being stage C (through capsule), or even stage D1 (lymph node metastases). Positive margins are especially likely if the tumor is large or the cells have a high Gleason score.

Many authorities recommend adding radiation therapy to radical prostatectomies that have positive margins. The rationale is that there are still left in the body cancer cells that need to be killed. This is adjuvant radiation therapy, which is also advocated by many doctors when the PSA value fails to drop to undetectable levels after surgery. This makes sense, because a persistent PSA following radical prostatectomy is equivalent to residual cancer.

Not everyone is convinced of the value of adjuvant radiation therapy for failed prostatectomy, because it has not consistently improved survival rates. But some doctors still believe it appropriate if the margins are positive, especially if the cells are aggressive. In any case, it does prolong the time before cancer returns, so the quality if not the quantity of patient life is enhanced. Most doctors agree that instituting adjuvant therapy as soon as positive margins are discovered is better than waiting for cancer to recur. Anyone pursuing adjuvant radiation therapy should be aware of possible side effects, including leg swelling, rectal damage, and urinary and/or stool incontinence.

Besides positive margins, another unfortunate occurrence in as many as a fifth of all operations, depending on whose statistics you read, is that the pelvic lymph nodes are examined by frozen section, found to be negative for cancer, the prostatectomy proceeds, and the permanent section later shows the lymph nodes to be positive. The result is that an operation designed solely to remove cancer confined to the prostate has been performed when the disease has already spread beyond the gland. That sounds awful, but it may not necessarily be. Some doctors believe there is a lot to be said for reducing the size of a tumor with an operation before beginning hormonal therapy for metastases. That may be even more appropriate if the lymph node metastases are microscopic. A few surgeons even proceed with radical prostatectomy if the frozen section shows only microscopic lymph node metastases of a low Gleason score (nonaggressive). This is a controversial issue and few surgeons are willing to recommend continuing surgery after a positive frozen section. Many do agree that the number of positive lymph nodes makes a difference. A cancer with microscopic metastases is preferable to one with a single positive lymph node, which is preferable to one with multiple positive nodes. Even more important is the grade (Gleason score) of the metastatic cancer cells; the worse the grade, the worse the prognosis.

Adjuvant hormonal therapy is usually appropriate when lymph node metastases are discovered after a radical prostatectomy. Like adjuvant radiation therapy, it does not prolong survival, only postpones the period before cancer reappears. Hormonal therapy is also indicated if the pathologist finds the cancer has spread to the seminal vesicles, because that usually means the tumor has metastasized to other organs.

Can Hormonal Therapy Shrink My Tumor Before Surgery?

Hormonal therapy given for several months can shrink the prostate gland. Therefore, some researchers have investigated whether this would make it easier to remove the entire gland. This method is neoadjuvant therapy, or endocrine downstaging. It is of special interest in stage C (through capsule) cancer, which is otherwise untreatable with surgery. It does shrink the tumor, but the tumor cells do not recede into the gland, so the situation itself is not improved.

Can Surgery Be Used if Radiation Fails?

Yes. This is salvage surgery and it follows situations where a biopsy shows persistent cancer 18 to 24 months after radiation therapy has been completed. But salvage prostatectomy is a more difficult procedure than standard prostatectomy, because the radiation causes inflammation and scar tissue formation that obliterates many of the anatomic landmarks the surgeon follows when performing the procedure. Complications, including incontinence, impotence, and rectal injury are more common than in nonsalvage operations.

Some surgeons feel salvage prostatectomy should not be performed, contending that hormonal therapy is the best salvage treatment. Others believe it is a reasonable procedure for certain men. Generally, anyone considering a salvage prostatectomy should have a minimum 10-year life expectancy, a negative bone scan, and seminal vesicles free of cancer. Experts do agree that surgery which requires adjuvant radiation therapy is a much easier path than radiation that results in salvage surgery. You and your doctor must consider the possibility of a future need for additional therapy when you make your primary therapy decision. Always plan ahead!

Are There New Types of Surgery Ahead?

Cryosurgical ablation is one new technique using liquid nitrogen to freeze cancer cells. Under ultrasound guidance, needles are inserted into the perineum, the area between the scrotum and anus. A thin probe is introduced through one of the needles into the prostate. Liquid nitrogen circulates through the probe (none actually entering the body), freezing the prostate. The physician can watch the prostate turn into an "ice ball" on ultrasound and turn off the machine when the procedure is complete.

The advantages of cryoablation are almost no bleeding, few complications, and you can go home the next day. The major disadvantage: it does not kill *all* of the cancer cells on the first try. Therefore, it is probably best used in older men or as a salvage procedure after failed radiation therapy. Cryoablation is experimental, but shows great promise.

Another cutting-edge form of experimental surgery is radioimmunoguided surgery (RIGS). In this technique, antibody molecules designed to bind to cancer cells are tagged with a radioactive label and injected into the body. These antibody molecules seek out cancer cells and attach to them. The surgeon then uses a hand-held radiation detector during surgery to identify areas of tumor spread. The same detector can be attached to the end of a laparoscope to zero in on positive nodes during lymph node dissection.

Increased understanding of prostate anatomy and cancer biology, major advancements in medical instrumentation and surgical techniques, and improvements in the operative skills of urologic surgeons have encouraged the popularity of surgery as a treatment for prostate cancer in recent years. Public awareness of radical prostatectomy as a cancer treatment greatly exceeds that of other forms of treatment. There are other treatments, of course, some far more appropriate than surgery in certain situations. To make an informed therapy decision, you must be well versed in all these options and realize that your choice among them depends on many factors. You must think of your disease as unique.

Chapter 6

What Is Radiation Therapy?

Radiation has been used for decades to treat prostate diseases. Radiation therapy bombards prostate tumors with radioactive energy in doses lethal to cancer cells. This radiation can be delivered in one of two ways—by external beam, also called teletherapy, or by interstitial implants, also referred to as brachytherapy.

Remember the last time you had an x-ray taken? The technician placed a film plate under the part of your anatomy to be examined and pointed an x-ray camera at it. The technician pushed a button and a beam of radiation traveled from the camera, through your body, and onto the film. External beam radiation therapy works much the same; the only difference is that doses of radiation required to kill cancers are a lot higher than what is needed to expose a piece of film. Because of these higher doses, holding still and focusing the beam accurately are much more important.

The machine that delivers external beam radiation therapy is a high-energy linear accelerator, and it emits radiation in discrete little "packets" of energy called photons. Radiation doses, both by external beams or interstitial implants, are measured in units abbreviated as *cGy* (or Gy, equal to 100 cGy). You may also hear the term *rad* used by radiation oncologists; it is the same as cGy. Doses for prostate cancer range from about 6000 cGy for a stage A1 tumor (small amount of cancer that cannot be felt) to over 7000 cGy for a stage C cancer (through capsule). These are high doses of radiation, so they must be spread out over six to seven weeks to decrease radiation toxicity. Because normal cells are also killed by radiation, your doctor must take great pains to make sure only a minimal amount of normal tissue is exposed to the radiation beam. No two radiation therapy regimens are exactly alike; each is tailored individually to match the stage and grade of your tumor, the shape and position of your prostate, and all the other qualities that make you unique.

The first step in radiation therapy is a planning stage called simulation, when the radiation oncologist customizes the area that will receive radiation according to your particular body and tumor. You will probably have to empty your bowels and retain your urine during simulation, because these maneuvers help to hold your prostate in the best position. You will also have a cast designed especially for you that will hold your body in exactly the same position for each radiation treatment, essential to ensure that the radiation always hits its mark.

Once you are immobilized and your bowels and bladder are appropriately empty and full, respectively, your doctor will perform a number of tests to pinpoint the target area. Special dye is inserted into the urethra and barium goes into the rectum so that these structures can be seen on x-ray. A CT scan is performed to locate the prostate and seminal vesicles. Knowing what the inside of your body looks like the oncologist can map out your individual treatment area to ensure that the radiation hits the cancer, not the surrounding normal tissue.

The intestines, anus, back wall of the rectum, and nonprostatic portions of the urethra are protected from the radiation beam by special shields called collimators. These prevent normal tissues from being irradiated and keep the beam traveling in a straight line, not bouncing off everybody else in the room. Collimators are custom-designed for you and your cancer, based upon the x-rays obtained during simulation.

Once simulation is complete, the actual therapy can begin. The first phase of treatment usually involves full-pelvic radiation, during which a generous portion of tissue surrounding the prostate is included in the field of radiation. The rationale is that microscopic amounts of cancer tissue often wander far from the original site. The external beam is aimed at the cancer from the top, bottom, and both sides to maximize coverage. Doses of approximately 200 cGy are given each day for about two weeks. After this initial stretch of full-pelvic radiation, the irradiated area is closed down to focus solely on the tumor. This is a cone-down booster dose and serves two functions: it gives the bowel and bladder a much-needed rest from radiation and guarantees the prostate will receive most of the total radiation dosage. The booster dose is given for about two weeks, then full-pelvic radiation is administered again for an additional two weeks or so. The total dose from start to finish ranges from 6500 to 7000 cGy, depending on the tumor's stage, with 2000 cGy given as a booster dose and the rest as full pelvic. The entire course of radiation treatment takes 6 to 7 weeks.

Paul G. was able to skip the full-pelvic phase of treatment and receive the cone-down booster alone, because he was over 75 and had a tumor with a very low Gleason score (nonaggressive). Clarence E. also received a booster dose by itself as an adjuvant to unsuccessful radical prostatectomy. Men with positive margins (cancer left behind) or who have a rising PSA within the first 18 months after surgery usually can be treated with a cone-down booster dose of radiation. Typically, men with a rising PSA more than 18 months after surgery require a full-pelvic dose.

External beam radiation therapy, like radical prostatectomy, has always been plagued by the fact that a substantial number of larger tumors cannot be cured and reappear after treatment. Radiation oncologists have tried for a long time to increase radiation doses enough to kill more cancer cells, but have only caused more side effects. Today, new technology allows physicians to focus radiation on tumors with far greater precision, thus increasing doses to the prostate while simultaneously decreasing doses to the normal tissues. The 3-D conformal technique uses computerized planning to make a three-dimensional image of your prostate so your oncologist can create more precise collimators and move them closer to your tumor, leaving just enough of an outside margin to allow for microscopic spread and the inevitable movement you might make during treatment. The margin can be made tighter over areas where movement or spread is less likely. The beam is then fired from six, not four, directions while an ultrasound device keeps track of the position of your prostate during treatment. The end result: increased dose to the tumor with reduced involvement of normal tissue. The 3-D conformal technique is relatively new and works best with smaller tumors with lower Gleason scores.

What Is Brachytherapy?

Brachytherapy, or interstitial implant therapy, involves the actual placement of radioactive material into the prostate itself. This treatment has been around since the beginning of the century, but advances in external beam technology during the 1980s caused the popularity of implants to decline significantly. However, the limits on external beam dosages, the high rate of cancer recurrences after treatment, and improvements in the accurate placement of implants have all led to renewed interest in brachytherapy in the 1990s.

Many different radioactive substances have been used in brachytherapy, including iodine (^{125}I), palladium (^{103}Pd), gold (^{198}Au), and iridium (^{192}Ir). The implants are inserted through needles that are placed in the perineum between the scrotum and anus. A rectangular plate with holes in it, a template, is placed against the perineum to assure accurate needle insertion. A CT scan confirms that the implants are in the prostate. The radioactive material is either removed after 48 to 60 hours, in the case of gold or iridium, or remains permanently, as with iodine or palladium.

With brachytherapy as salvage therapy after failed surgery or external beam radiation, implant placement can be done under transrectal ultrasound (TRUS). When done as the primary therapeutic modality, a pelvic lymph node dissection (PLND) is usually done at the same time, because radiation therapy will not cure cancer that has metastasized. If the frozen section is positive, the procedure is ended; if negative, implantation proceeds. The surgeon helps by holding the prostate while the oncologist places the needles and implants into the gland guided by the template. Today, this entire procedure can usually be performed laparoscopically.

Brachytherapy can be used in a variety of situations, including by itself for tumors completely contained within the prostate (stage B1, for example). But experts agree brachytherapy alone is not nearly as effective as external beam therapy alone, because dosage uniformity is inferior. The more common use of interstitial implants and the one you are most likely to encounter is used in conjunction with external beam radiation, because it allows an increase in the total dose of radiation without increasing the exposure of normal tissues. External beam radiation typically is given first, then after a two-to-three week rest period, brachytherapy is administered. A newer technique involves giving brachytherapy first, then following with external beam.

The advantages of brachytherapy are obvious. The therapy duration is much shorter—the prefix "brachy" means "short"—than with external beam, with total length of hospitalization ranging from four to ten days (or less when TRUS is used). The implants deliver concentrated doses of radiation to the tumor while sparing the surrounding tissue, thus reducing side effects. PLND can be done at the same time rather than as a separate procedure, as with external beam therapy. Brachytherapy is a reasonable choice for men like Harold H., who had a small, nonaggressive tumor and multiple medical problems that made him a poor surgical risk. It also is appropriate for men like Oscar A. and Francis G., who suffered recurrences of their tumors after radical prostatectomy and external beam radiation therapy, respectively. Brachytherapy is not available everywhere, though, so you should discuss this and other options with your oncologist.

What Is Hyperthermia?

Hyperthermia means "excessive temperature" and it has been used for some time as an experimental form of treatment for relieving painful inflammatory and obstructive prostate conditions. Not until recently has this technology found a role in treating prostate cancer. Physicians have discovered that heating the prostate kills cancer cells, increases your immune system's ability to kill cancer cells, enhances the effect that radiation and chemotherapy drugs have on tumor cells, and relieves many of the uncomfortable symptoms of metastatic disease like urinary obstruction and pelvic pain. Some men with widespread disease have actually enjoyed a regression (shrinking) of their metastases, because of the immune-system stimulation that hyperthermia elicits.

The two most commonly used instruments for delivering hyperthermic therapy to the prostate are microwaves and electrodes. The microwave technique utilizes a probe inserted into the rectum; water-cooling protects the rectum from heat damage. The prostate is heated to as high as 45°C (113°F) for about one hour. This is done six to ten times over the course of one to two weeks. Electrodes typically are used in conjunction with brachytherapy and are inserted through the perineal template in the same way as the radioactive implants. Electrical current is applied to the electrodes and the prostate is heated for about 45 minutes. The procedure does cause some pain, especially when the seminal vesicles are heated, but it can be controlled with medication. Hyperthermia treatments are usually given immediately before and immediately after implantation and enhance the sensitivity of the cancer cells to the radiation. Hyperthermic therapy is not widespread.

What Are the Side Effects of Radiation Therapy?

As you might expect, most radiation side effects stem from its effect on normal tissue. Exposed areas of the rectum can become inflamed, leading to pain, bleeding, and ulcers. Scar tissue may cause the rectum to constrict at certain points. Similar effects occur on the urinary tract, with bladder inflammation, bloody urine, and urethral constriction the most common. Severe complications, like rectal damage that necessitate a colostomy, urinary incontinence, and fistulae (abnormal tubelike communications) between the rectum and urinary tract, are fortunately less frequent. As with surgery, these are rare complications.

Undoubtedly, the complication you are most interested in is impotence, unfortunately a common side effect of radiation therapy, with a frequency that ranges from 14 to 50 percent, depending on age, other medical problems, and pretreatment sexual function. The risk of impotence is significantly less with brachytherapy (4–10 percent) than with external beam therapy, one of the primary advantages of the former. The other potential complications of brachytherapy are similar but less frequent than external beam, with urinary obstruction the most common. Side effects tend to be at their worst about two months after implantation, with gradual improvement afterward.

When Is Adjuvant or Palliative Radiation Appropriate?

In the previous chapter, we briefly discussed adjuvant therapy, supplemental treatment given to a tumor when the primary therapy choice doesn't kill all the cancer cells. Don't confuse this with salvage therapy, treatment not given until recurrence of a previously treated cancer is identified. Adjuvant radiation is usually prescribed when positive margins or seminal vesicle involvement is noted during a radical prostatectomy. These cases are at a high risk for metastases to the pelvic lymph nodes, so the nodes are usually included in the radiation field. Radiation also can be used as an adjuvant to radiation—brachytherapy when external beam is the primary treatment and external beam when brachytherapy is the primary.

Isaac M. had metastatic prostate cancer that would not respond to treatment and his doctor wanted to make his remaining time as comfortable as possible. The growth of the tumor was causing many disturbing and painful symptoms, such as rectal and pelvic pain, urinary obstruction, and leg swelling. He also had extremely painful metastases to the bones of his vertebral column. Fortunately, he was able to avoid compression of the spinal cord, which happens to many men with metastatic disease and is a medical emergency that causes leg pain, weakness, sensory loss, urinary retention, and incontinence. Nevertheless, he was still in a great deal of distress.

Isaac's doctor prescribed palliative radiation therapy, meaning there was no chance for cure, and treatment was purely for symptomatic relief. Palliative radiation is usually delivered by external beam, but radioactive substances, like strontium (^{89}Sr), phosphorus (^{32}P), or rhenium (^{186}Re), can be injected into the body to give widespread coverage when the metastases are too numerous to treat with a beam.

What If I Have Cancer Remaining After My Radiation Therapy?

If you could obtain biopsies from every man who had just completed radiation therapy for prostate cancer, most of those biopsies would be positive, because one consequence of prostatic carcinoma's being a slow-growing cancer is that it also is a slow-*dying* cancer. It can take a full 18 to 24 months for the final effect of the radiation on the tumor cells to become evident. Meanwhile, the prostate is populated by countless radiation-damaged cells that look a lot like cancer to all but the most specially trained pathologists. This has led to a heated debate among experts as to who should have biopsies after radiation therapy and what should be done if they prove positive.

A man with a positive biopsy can live for 15 years even as a man with a negative biopsy can experience rapid progression of his disease. But men with positive post-treatment biopsies generally have a higher risk of cancer recurrence than those with negative biopsies. Most experts agree it is unnecessary for everyone to have a biopsy after radiation therapy, especially since the advent of prostate specific antigen (PSA). Your doctor will undoubtedly follow your PSA levels for many years after radiation therapy, because that is the best way to detect a recurrence early. If the PSA moves in the wrong direction, a biopsy clearly is indicated. A biopsy is also appropriate if your doctor feels some abnormality during a digital rectal exam (DRE). If the biopsy in these situations is positive, adjuvant therapy (i.e., hormonal) should be considered. The sooner after initial radiation treatment that a positive PSA, DRE, or biopsy change occurs, the worse the prognosis.

The risk of recurrence or metastasis after radiation therapy depends greatly on the stage and grade of the tumor before treatment. A localized stage (A and B), a low Gleason score (nonaggressive), and a low pretreatment PSA level all suggest a good possibility of successful treatment. On the other hand, an advanced stage (C), a high Gleason score (aggressive), and a high PSA reading signify a poor prognosis and adjuvant hormonal therapy might be necessary. Carl S. knew that he had a high risk of eventually developing metastases when his tumor caused urethral obstruction to the point where a transurethral resection (TURP) was required to relieve symptoms. Curiously, older men usually have a *lower* risk of metastasis than younger men, because their tumors are usually less aggressive. Any man who has had radiation therapy has a finite risk of recurrence that lasts as long as 15 years, so you should continue to see your doctor at regular intervals for this entire period.

How Do I Decide If Radiation Is Right for Me?

In the previous chapter, we mentioned the great debate that surrounds the need for and the choice of prostate cancer therapy. The hottest issue is surgery vs. radiation in treating stage A and B (confined to the prostate) carcinomas. Urologists claim surgery is superior and radiation oncologists believe radiation is better, and they both have evidence to back their arguments. How can they both be right?

If you look only at survival statistics, you will see that overall survival figures are better for surgery than for radiation provided the tumor is confined to the prostate. However, as with many things in life, the facts are not that simple. Surgery has better numbers because men who are fit enough to undergo radical prostatectomy are generally younger and healthier than most radiation patients. When the playing field is leveled by taking age and health into account, surgery and radiation are equally effective treatments. Similarly, surgery and radiation are equally *ineffective* treatments for metastatic disease (stage D). That remains the domain of hormonal therapy.

Most doctors agree radiation is the best choice for stage C (through capsule) carcinoma of the prostate. Even so, a man with stage C disease has at best a 50-50 chance to live 10 years after radiation therapy, because microscopic metastases are more the rule than the exception in such cases. There is a lot of room for improvement in medicine's ability to treat cancer that has extended beyond the prostate. Radiation is the preferred choice for tumors too large or too aggressive to be amenable to prostatectomy. Adjuvant or neoadjuvant hormonal therapy can be added to the treatment plan to shrink large tumors to a convenient size for radiation therapy.

Anything New in Radiation Therapy?

One of the most active areas in radiation therapy research is the use of particles in radiation beams. Instead of firing photons (which have no mass) at a tumor, subatomic particles called fast neutrons are used. These allow up to 100 times the energy to be delivered to cancer cells, translating into more dead cells and a better result. The main drawback of fast-neutron beams is their higher rate of complications, which has led some scientists to combine the neutrons and photons into a mixed beam, which has the best of both worlds. There is more work to be done before fast neutrons are widely accepted, but the technology may eventually replace what is in use today.

Radiation therapy remains one of the primary treatment methods for prostate tumors that have the potential for being cured. Along with radical prostatectomy, it will be used for many years. Neither method is likely to usurp the other anytime soon. Age, stage, grade, and many other factors will determine which is better for you. Cancer that has advanced beyond the curable stage falls into the realm of hormonal therapy, covered in the next chapter.

Chapter 7

What Is Hormonal Therapy?

Now that we are considering hormonal therapy, our discussion will take on a decidedly different tone than with surgery or radiation, because many of the men for whom surgery or radiation are prescribed to treat their cancers have a realistic chance to be cured of their disease. Unfortunately, that cannot be said about those who receive hormonal therapy. If you and your doctor have selected hormonal manipulation as your primary treatment method, you probably have metastatic cancer and your main goal is to diminish the effects not cure your disease. This lack of curative potential explains why hormones are not used as primary therapy in nonmetastatic cancer.

If there is anything positive about your having metastatic prostate cancer, it is that you are not alone. From 25 to 50 percent of all men diagnosed with prostate cancer have metastatic disease when diagnosed. Even men who are told they have only stage B (confined to gland) or C (through capsule) tumors end up having lymph node metastases (stage D1) 20–40 percent of the time, and 85 percent of the time these nodal metastases spread to the bone (stage D2) within five years. The average survival of men with metastatic prostate cancer is only about 24 to 30 months, and only 20 percent of them survive five years. To make matters worse, hormonal therapy does not change any of these survival figures.

No doubt this all sounds terribly ominous, but it does not mean you have to quit. Hormonal therapy cannot cure prostatic carcinoma, but it can do a lot to alleviate the symptoms of metastatic cancer and to extend the amount of time that you can live a productive life without constantly being made aware of the presence of a tumor within you. Put another way, hormonal therapy is designed to improve the quality of your remaining time, if not its quantity. As many as 80–85 percent of the men who receive hormonal therapy derive some benefit, including tumor shrinkage, urinary obstruction relief, decreased bone pain, anemia reversal, reduction in PSA level, and improved appetite.

How Does Hormonal Therapy Work?

Back in chapters 1 and 2, we learned the prostate gland depends on the male hormone testosterone for normal growth and function. Testosterone is one of several hormones in the category of *androgens*, the hormones responsible for male physical traits like muscle mass, body hair, and deep voice. Unfortunately, androgens not only fuel the growth of normal prostate cells, they exert an identical effect on prostate cancer cells. The rationale behind hormonal therapy is to block that connection between androgens and the tumor.

Testosterone secretion by the testes is controlled by the pituitary gland, which hangs from the bottom of your brain like a pea-sized punching bag. The pituitary is controlled by a portion of the brain called the hypothalamus, which stimulates the pituitary by secreting luteinizing hormone-releasing hormone (LHRH), causing the pituitary to produce luteinizing hormone (LH). LH signals the testes to release testosterone. When it reaches the prostate, testosterone is converted to its more active form dihydrotestosterone (DHT), with the help of a prostatic chemical called 5-α-reductase, (Figure 7-1).

Hormonal therapy interrupts these pathways at various points, depriving the tumor of the androgens it needs. A problem with this strategy is that androgens are also produced by another set of glands, the adrenals, resting atop the kidneys. The hypothalamus also secretes corticotrophin-releasing hormone (CRH), which causes the pituitary to release adrenocorticotropic hormone (ACTH), which signals the adrenals to produce androgens. These adrenal-manufactured androgens can continue to feed cancer cells even when testicular androgens are blocked with hormonal therapy.

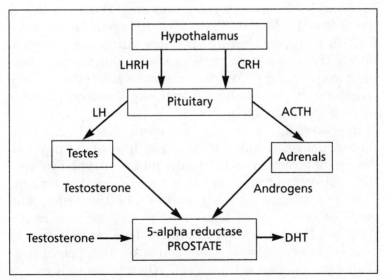

Figure 7.1: The Influence of Androgens on the Prostate

What Are the Varieties of Hormonal Therapy?

The method of removing testicular androgens that has stood the test of time is castration, or orchiectomy. While the mere thought of surgical removal of the testes frightens most men, there is a lot to be said for this therapy in metastatic cancer cases. It is considerably less expensive than many of the drugs used in hormonal therapy and works very rapidly, in 12 hours or less in most instances. Orchiectomy has another advantage over drugs: you don't need to remember to take your pills.

If your doctor has recommended orchiectomy, it is perfectly understandable for you to be concerned. Many men worry about the physiologic effects testicular removal will have on them and also about what their bodies will look like after the surgery. Impotence and loss of sexual desire occur with almost every orchiectomy. That was not a major issue for Marvin B., who was impotent for years before his treatment, but if it is important to you, let your doctor know so he can consider your feelings when planning your therapy. Another common side effect of orchiectomy is "hot flashes" resembling those experienced by menopausal women.

Improvements in surgical technique should help your urologist alleviate any fears you may have about physical deformities from an orchiectomy. Subcapsular and subepididymal orchiectomies are new techniques that remove only testosterone-secreting portions of the testes, but leave behind enough tissue so the scrotum can retain its shape. These are not yet routinely done by urologic surgeons, however, so make sure you know the type of procedure your doctor will perform. When you review everything, you will appreciate that orchiectomy is an inexpensive, simple method of hormonal therapy that achieves rapid results with minimal side effects.

Among the first drugs used for hormonal treatment of prostate cancer were estrogens, female hormones. The most commonly used was diethylstilbestrol (DES), very effective in blocking the secretion of LH by the pituitary, thus removing the primary means by which the testes are stimulated into producing testosterone. DES has been around for a long time and is inexpensive. Even so, DES is not used much today, because it causes substantial side effects, some serious. Nausea and vomiting, fluid retention and swelling, impotence and loss of sex drive, headaches, disorders of protein and fat metabolism, and breast growth are some of the less dangerous effects of DES therapy. Some of the potentially fatal reactions include heart attack, stroke, and lower extremity blood clots, which can break off and lodge in the lungs. There are safer, more effective drugs available now, so DES has almost become obsolete for treating prostate cancer.

Estrogens are the female equivalent of male androgens and are responsible for development of sexual characteristics in women. Women also produce another class of hormones called progestins that support their wombs during pregnancy. Like estrogens, progestins have a role in treating metastatic prostate cancer. Megestrol (MGA) (Megace®) and Cyproterone (CPA) are the progestins used most frequently in prostate cancer, although the latter is not FDA-approved in the U.S. Progestins exert two effects simultaneously to block the effects of androgens on prostate cancer. First, they prevent androgens from attaching to the tumor, and second, they block pituitary LH secretion. Unlike estrogens, they do not cause serious heart side effects. Unfortunately, that is probably their only advantage. A profound disadvantage of progestins is that they stop working after six to nine months and the testosterone level begins to rise again.

Progestins are also referred to as steroidal antiandrogens, because their chemical structure resembles steroid hormones produced by the adrenal glands. Their counterpart, nonsteroidal antiandrogens, are some of the newest drugs available for hormonal therapy. Nonsteroidal antiandrogens prevent binding of testosterone and DHT to their targets, but do not prevent formation of these androgens, so blood levels of testosterone and DHT remain high. This is very significant, because it means potency and sexual desire can be preserved!

The only nonsteroidal antiandrogen used in the U.S. at this writing is flutamide (Eulexin®); another, Casodex®, is expected to be approved soon. Flutamide side effects include diarrhea, flushing, and breast growth. The only potentially serious side effect is liver toxicity, which is rare and usually reversible. Undoubtedly, the most significant drawback to nonsteroidal antiandrogens is their extremely high price tag. Flutamide therapy can cost $300 or more *per month*, a serious consideration unless your insurance plan defrays the cost.

No nonsteroidal antiandrogen is approved in the U.S. for use by itself. The FDA has approved them only in combination with an orchiectomy or with a member of the newest class of drugs, the luteinizing hormone-releasing hormone (LHRH) agonists. We will discuss this combination later. LHRH agonists essentially perform surgery without cutting by effecting a medical, rather than a surgical, castration. The net result is identical to orchiectomy, but the testes remain. These drugs take the place of your own LHRH, initially stimulating your pituitary into secreting increased amounts of LH. When the gland soon becomes unresponsive to stimulation, LH production plummets and the testes no longer release testosterone.

Because LH secretion rises before it falls is probably the most troublesome effect of LHRH agonists. Increased LH leads to increased androgens, which means more fuel for the tumor and exacerbated symptoms. In other words, the very thing you are trying to improve with hormonal therapy instead is (temporarily) made worse. This initial worsening of symptoms is called the "flare effect" and is characteristic of LHRH agonists. Fortunately, the flare effect can be avoided by administering an antiandrogen such as flutamide for a brief period. Once the LH level falls, the antiandrogen can be stopped.

The two LHRH agonists that are currently in use in the U.S. are leuprolide (Lupron®) and goserelin (Zoladex®). Both drugs are available in depot forms, long-lasting injections that need to be given only once a month, which is a tremendous convenience, because you can travel and enjoy your life without being tied down to your medical therapy. The side effects are similar to other drug classes, with impotence, hot flashes, loss of sex drive, fluid retention, breast growth, and injection site irritation the most common. LHRH agonists, like nonsteroidal antiandrogens, are new and therefore very expensive. Goserelin runs slightly more than $300 a month, while leuprolide costs over $400 a month. All these hormonal therapy agents are listed in Table 7.1.

How Do You Block Androgens from the Adrenal Glands?

Earlier, we mentioned that androgens are produced not only by the testes, but also by the adrenal glands. When testicular androgens are blocked or removed with hormonal therapy, adrenal androgens remain in the bloodstream and can stimulate the growth of prostate cancer.

Table 7.1
Different Forms of Hormonal Therapy

---

1. Orchiectomy (castration)
2. Estrogens
   a. Diethylstilbestrol (DES)
   b. Estramustine
   c. Polyestradiol
3. Steroidal Antiandrogens (Progestins)
   a. Cyproterone (CPA)*
   b. Medroxyprogesterone
   c. Megestrol (MGA) (Megace®)
4. Nonsteroidal Antiandrogens
   a. Flutamide (Eulexin®)
   b. Nilutamide (Anandron®)*
   c. Casodex®*
5. LHRH Agonists
   a. Leuprolide (Lupron®)
   b. Goserelin (Zoladex®)
   c. Buserelin*
6. Steroid Synthesis Blockers
   a. Ketoconazole (Nizoral®)
   b. Aminoglutethimide
   c. Spironolactone (Aldactone®)

*Not approved by the FDA for use in the U.S.

This adrenal contribution makes up only about 5–10 percent of androgens in the blood, but composes 25–40 percent of androgens within the prostate, which is more important. This effect has generated a lot of interest in finding methods to block adrenal as well as testicular androgens.

A drug category that has been used to accomplish this function is the steroid synthesis blockers. As their name implies, they actually prevent manufacture of steroid hormones and androgens. They include aminoglutethimide, traditionally used for seizure disorders, spironolactone (Aldactone®), a diuretic that manages fluid accumulation and high blood pressure, and ketoconazole (Nizoral®), an antifungal. These agents have not been used much in hormonal therapy, however, because they have many side effects, do not work well, and do not work for long. Ketoconazole is probably the only drug utilized semi-consistently, and then only in emergencies like spinal cord compression or severe blood clotting abnormalities. In these circumstances, ketoconazole works very well because its effects occur rapidly. It is a good drug for men who, for one reason or another, cannot have an orchiectomy. Kenneth P.'s doctor prescribed ketoconazole for him to prevent the flare effects from the LHRH agonist he was taking. Ketoconazole side effects include loss of sexual desire, weakness, liver inflammation, dry mouth, and adrenal gland suppression.

A more effective and more widely used option for blocking testicular and adrenal androgens is to use an antiandrogen like flutamide, along with an LHRH agonist or an orchiectomy. This strategy of combining drugs is called total androgen blockade and it is very controversial. Those who favor it claim it actually prolongs survival by 7 to 15 months, especially when tumors are less widespread. Doctors who oppose the therapy state it does not enhance survival and, therefore, its extremely high cost is unjustified. The cost can be lowered by choosing an orchiectomy over the LHRH agonist, but this still does not address whether total androgen blockade really works. The answer will not be available anytime soon, because this type of hormonal therapy is very new. Therefore, what you do with this information will depend on your situation and your doctor's treatment philosophy. Some men would rather not take an expensive drug with serious side effects unless it has been proven. Others, faced with metastatic cancer that will eventually kill them, are willing to try anything with even a remote possibility of helping. You must decide for yourself.

A less controversial use of total androgen blockade is in a neoadjuvant capacity before radiation therapy occurs. As we learned in the previous chapter, hormonal therapy is administered to shrink the tumor to a more manageable size before radiation is delivered. Leuprolide and flutamide are given for three months before radiation therapy, causing the tumor to become more sharply separated from surrounding normal tissues. Neoadjuvant hormonal therapy does not work well for radical prostatectomy, but is quite useful as a lead-in to radiation therapy.

Should I Start Therapy Now or Wait for Symptoms to Develop?

The controversy surrounding hormonal therapy does not end with total androgen blockade. The debate over early versus delayed therapy is equally passionate and significant, and there are convincing arguments on both sides. Those supporting initiation of therapy as soon as metastatic cancer is diagnosed claim it improves the quality of remaining life because therapy postpones the onset of bothersome and painful symptoms. Early therapy was not often used in the past because the older drugs (i.e., DES) had many side effects. Newer, safer drugs have made early therapy more realistic. Wayne P. opted for early therapy because he did not want to sit around doing nothing while waiting for his tumor to advance.

Those who believe it is better to wait until symptoms appear before prescribing hormonal therapy maintain that giving expensive, potentially toxic drugs to a man without symptoms is not prudent, especially when this type of therapy has never proved to increase survival. They say the side effects outweigh the benefits and that the results are the same if you wait for symptoms to appear. In fact, men who defer hormonal therapy often have more energy and fewer sexual difficulties. Again, we have an unresolved issue! As before, your final decision will depend on your situation and your doctor's treatment philosophy.

How Long Is Hormonal Therapy Effective?

Hormonal therapy can accomplish a remission in prostate cancer, not a cure. Symptoms are suppressed and quality of life is improved for a finite period, but eventually the cancer becomes resistant to this treatment. This is called escape, or relapse, and occurs sooner or later in almost every case of metastatic disease. Most experts think the heterogeneous nature (different cell types in the same tumor) of prostatic carcinoma allows it to relapse. Hormonal therapy is effective in treating androgen-dependent cells within the tumor. However, every tumor also has a population of androgen-independent cells that continue to multiply despite therapy. This androgen-independent component is ultimately fatal. Relapse can occur anytime, from 6 to 18 months after initiating hormonal therapy. Once the tumor escapes, additional hormonal therapy is useless, because only androgen-independent cells remain. Half of all men die within six months when they reach the hormone-unresponsive stage (D3) of prostate cancer.

The prostate-specific antigen (PSA) level can help assess the androgen-dependent and -independent qualities of a tumor, which can help determine your likelihood of responding to hormonal therapy. Androgen-dependent cells produce larger amounts of PSA than their androgen-independent counterparts. If hormonal therapy causes your PSA level to drop into the range of normal, your tumor probably has a significant androgen-dependent component and your response to therapy will likely be good. On the contrary, if your PSA level remains elevated despite hormonal therapy, your response to treatment will probably be poor. An increase in PSA after an initial decrease signifies a relapse. We already know the PSA reading is only one of many tools needed to evaluate tumor status. The digital rectal exam and bone scan are also essential for getting the full picture.

What Can I Do If My Tumor Won't Respond to Hormones?

Neil J. developed stage D3 (hormone-unresponsive) disease shortly after receiving total androgen blockade therapy with flutamide and an LHRH agonist. The first thing his doctor did was stop the flutamide, causing Neil's PSA level to drop and improving his painful symptoms. A number of chemotherapy drugs have been used in prostate cancer: vinblastine, trimetrexate, mitoguazone, doxurubicin, epirubicin, and estramustine are all poisonous to cancer cells. But these agents have many side effects, including heart failure, bone marrow suppression, and hair loss, and they have had pitifully low success rates in the treatment of prostate cancer. In fact, most experts believe chemotherapy has no place at all in prostate cancer therapy.

That leaves clinical trials as the final treatment option for metastatic prostate carcinoma that no longer responds to hormonal therapy. New treatment methods are continually being investigated in research centers, and the physicians who conduct this research always need volunteers to test their cutting-edge ideas. Thousands of men with prostate cancer enlist in these studies each year, because they feel they have nothing to lose. If you are interested in trying an experimental treatment, ask your doctor if he knows about any current clinical trials and if you would be eligible.

Chapter 8

When Should You or Should You Not Intervene?

So far, the story of prostate cancer has been controversy after controversy. The greatest of all is in this chapter: whether to treat prostate cancer *at all*. Many physicians, scientists, ethicists, and patient advocates argue that because prostate cancer is a slow-growing disease that occurs in elderly men and progresses despite any attempts to treat it, leaving it alone and addressing any symptoms as they arise is a legitimate therapy option. This argument has considerable merit. But, first, let's review the natural history of how a normal prostate gland becomes cancerous, and at what point during this transformation should the problem be identified and corrected, if ever.

What Comes Between Normal and Cancerous Prostate?

In chapter 2, we learned prostate cancer is a malignant growth of abnormal cells that can take over the entire gland and spread to other organs. No man goes to sleep one night with a healthy prostate and awakens the next morning with cancer. Obviously, something happens between these extremes. Two types of prostate cell abnormalities are considered premalignant, meaning they occur somewhere between normal prostate and cancer. These changes are atypical adenomatous hyperplasia (AAH) and prostatic intraepithelial neoplasia (PIN).

With AAH, small, round, uniform, tightly packed glandular units (acini) with tiny excretory ducts branch off normal, pre-existing ducts. Viewed through a microscope, AAH looks like nonaggressive (low Gleason score) cancer. The main difference between cancer and AAH is that AAH cells appear normal, but are not completely normal because they are clustered together abnormally. AAH occurs mainly in the central zone of the prostate, which, as we know, is an uncommon location for cancer. When AAH is found on a biopsy or during a transurethral resection (TURP) for benign prostatic enlargement (BPH), it deserves to be watched closely, because it often means cancer is lurking somewhere else within the gland.

PIN is different from AAH, not only because it occurs in the peripheral zone of the prostate, the preferred location for cancer, but also because the cells themselves look more like cancer cells than normal cells. PIN cells are irregularly shaped with irregular spaces between them, and the inner workings of the cells are abnormally dark and enlarged. In fact, the only difference between cancer and PIN is that PIN does not extend through the basal cell layer that lines the ducts and acini like a barricade. When PIN does acquire the ability to break through this barrier, there is nothing left to prevent its spreading thoughout the gland and into other organs. This is how a premalignant condition like PIN becomes cancer; over 50 percent of prostate cancers evolve from PIN. Once PIN disrupts the basal cell layer, it allows PSA to escape from the gland and into the blood circulation. Therefore, PIN usually causes a PSA reading somewhere between BPH and cancer.

The closer PIN gets to crossing the basal cell layer, the higher the grade assigned to it. Grade 1 PIN is only slightly abnormal and can be observed over time for any changes, grade 2 PIN usually warrants periodic biopsies, while grade 3 PIN, called carcinoma in situ, tells your doctor bona fide cancer probably exists somewhere else within the same gland. If your doctor finds grade 3 PIN in your prostate after a biopsy or TURP, undoubtedly he will perform a repeat biopsy to look for cancer. If the second biopsy is negative, he will continue to follow you with frequent PSA tests and digital rectal exams. Any case of PIN associated with elevated PSA deserves a biopsy, regardless of grade. Generally, PIN does not itself signify a need for aggressive treatment, only aggressive observation.

Why Are Some Tumors Bad and Others Not So Bad?

We now know the pivotal event that transforms premalignant cells into malignant is their acquisition of the ability to cross the basal cell layer and invade the rest of the gland. As we discussed in chapter 2, this transformation occurs in most men once they reach a certain age. Many men carry cancerous tissue in their prostates, yet for most of them it is of no consequence. Therefore, there must be some factor that determines which tumors will grow slowly and cause no problems and which will grow rapidly and become lethal.

Cancer cells reproduce more rapidly than normal cells, with higher-grade (Gleason score) cells having a faster multiplication rate than lower grades. Each time a cell divides, there is a finite risk that the genetic material within it will mutate, giving it an entirely new identity. Cancer cells, because they divide more often, are at a greater risk of mutation than normal cells. Many experts believe all prostate cancers begin as small, low-grade tumors that remain nonaggressive until a mutation occurs during cell division, starting a whole new family of aggressive cells. That most prostate cancers are inconsequential suggests that this transforming mutation must be rare. The risk increases as the tumor grows, because more cells are available to mutate. The new high-grade cells proliferate rapidly and metastasize.

This is not the only theory that explains the source of aggressive tumors. Another suggests that high-grade tumors are aggressive from the very beginning when they evolve from high-grade PIN, explaining why some small tumors have high Gleason scores. These theories are *not* mutually exclusive. Some aggressive tumors probably do begin as low-grade cancer and mutate, while others are probably high-grade from their inception. No one knows which percentages of each exist.

Why is any of this of interest to you? If you have an early cancer that will require mutation to become high-grade, you will probably enjoy a normal life expectancy with or without treatment. If you have an early tumor that was high-grade from the beginning, you will probably fare poorly with or without treatment. In other words: THOSE WHO DO (WELL/POORLY), DO SO REGARDLESS OF TREATMENT. That is the heart of the argument of those adhering to the "watch-and-wait" philosophy. They believe the results achieved by men with prostate cancer depend not on the treatment, but on the tumor itself—high grade means poor prognosis; low grade means good prognosis.

When Is Watching-and-Waiting Appropriate?

As men live longer and screening tests like PSA and transrectal ultrasound (TRUS) are used with greater frequency, more and more new prostate cancers will be detected sooner each year. Many of these tumors will be very small and pose no danger to the men who have them. While many patients have asked what should be done about such tumors, more than a few doctors have suggested nothing be done at all. Prostate cancer grows slowly and occurs in older men, which means most of them die from causes other than their cancer (*with* cancer, not *from* it). Further, no one has ever proved that treating prostate cancer improves life expectancy at all. Radical prostatectomy and radiation therapy are popular treatment options, because technical improvements have significantly decreased their side effects, but neither has substantially affected the death rate from prostate cancer. Therefore, watching-and-waiting makes a great deal of sense when you consider the facts.

Watching-and-waiting is a less controversial strategy when applied to microscopic cancer discovered incidentally during a TURP for BPH (stage A1). Only 5 percent of men with stage A1 disease die within 10 years. The only problem with assigning a diagnosis of stage A1 cancer on the basis of a TURP is that this procedure removes tissue mainly from the periurethral and transition zones, and we know cancer is usually found in the peripheral zone. It is essential to make sure A1 cancer is not actually A2, because A2 has a 20 percent higher mortality rate. Any stage A1 cancer should be restaged with a biopsy or a repeat TURP. If no more cancer is found, periodic PSA tests and rectal exams are sufficient monitors. If additional cancer is found, then definitive therapy like surgery or radiation may be needed.

No debate is ever one-sided. Quite a few physicians distrust watching-and-waiting, contending that a significant number of tumors are too small to be felt, but may still be aggressive and able to spread beyond the prostate. They argue that while the chance for cure with radiation therapy or surgery may be small, it is preferable to the zero chance with no treatment. The only potential for cure exists with early-stage disease; watching-and-waiting allows the cancer to progress to a stage where cure is no longer possible. Even though it isn't necessary for your prostate cancer to be cured for you to live 10 years or more, these are still valid statements.

When your doctor is helping you plan your choice of prostate cancer therapy, he is obligated to list all legitimate options, including doing nothing. This is difficult for him, because if you fare poorly, both of you will wonder whether surgery or radiation would have made a difference. Watching-and-waiting is a reasonable treatment option if you are in your 70s or older and have an early cancer of a low or intermediate Gleason score. However, basing a treatment decision purely on a perceived lifespan is difficult. Males born in the U.S. have a 72-year life expectancy, but those who actually reach this age usually can look forward to another 10 years. Stanley T. interpreted his doctor's suggestion that they merely observe his tumor over time as physician abandonment. His doctor reassured him that was not the case at all and he still wanted to see Stanley at frequent intervals to follow the progression of his disease and to intervene with TURP or hormonal therapy if symptoms should arise.

Choosing watching-and-waiting (or any other treatment option) is not easy. You have to decide between a definitive treatment that may cause serious complications, cost a lot of money, and not prolong your life at all or a conservative strategy that offers no chance of cure and will almost certainly lead to metastases. Many men need help making such a crucial decision, so you may want to discuss with your doctor the possibility of bringing a social worker or psychologist into the planning process. These professionals are trained to balance important life issues like age, family, religion, and finances and can help relieve you of some of the decision-making burden.

The important thing to remember is that all men are not created equal. While watching-and-waiting may be fine for a man who is old and sick, it is far less appropriate for young, otherwise healthy men with many years ahead of them. No two men are alike and no two cancers are either, which reinforces the importance of frank, in-depth communication between you and your doctor to decide what is best for you.

Chapter 9

Can Prostate Cancer Be Prevented?

The previous four chapters were devoted to various treatments for prostatic carcinoma like surgery, radiation, hormonal therapy, and watchful waiting. Now, we will address prostate cancer prevention, a concept in its infancy and still being studied. Treatment and prevention sound as if they would be related, but are as different as apples and oranges. Let's look at some of those differences.

The purpose of any treatment method is to kill or remove cancer cells. Treatment is considered successful if the tumor is eradicated and you can live longer without cancer inside you. Unlike treatment, prevention strategies are aimed at a much earlier phase in cancer development. The goal of prevention is to block carcinogenesis, the step-by-step transformation of normal cells into cancerous ones. When prevention is successful, it stops cancer from developing in the first place. An effective prostate cancer prevention program would lead to a decrease in the number of new cases of the disease being diagnosed each year (incidence) and in the annual death rate (mortality). As an additional benefit of blocking carcinogenesis, a prevention program would also reduce the occurrence of PIN and AAH, the precancer changes we discussed in the previous chapter, and stave off progression of nonaggressive cells into aggressive ones.

Obviously, prevention and treatment are intended for two entirely different groups of individuals. Treatment is designed for people who've been diagnosed with a disease by their physicians. Prevention, on the other hand, is meant for those who have yet to develop the disease and don't want to get it. The latter can occur in a variety of settings, depending on the desired result. Some preventive measures, such as polio vaccines, are administered to the general population. Others, such as cholesterol-lowering drugs, are given only to people with an increased risk for acquiring coronary artery disease. Scientists are now studying several agents that may one day be used to prevent prostate cancer, but they have yet to decide what will be chosen and who should receive it. Most likely, men who eventually receive preventive therapy will be those at increased risk of developing cancer. These would include black men, men with a family history of prostate cancer, men with PIN or AAH, men with very early cancers who want to impede tumor growth, or men with previously treated cancers who want to avoid a recurrence.

Prostate cancer seems the ideal disease to become the target of a prevention program. It grows slowly and there is a long interval between when the tumor is small and nonaggressive and when it is large and aggressive, thus providing an ample window of opportunity when preventive therapy can be employed. Prostatic carcinoma is unique because of its high number of microscopic cancers. As we know, once most men reach a certain age, they have some degree of cancer in their prostates. Preventive agents could block those tumors from progressing to a dangerous stage. Most important is that treatment for many prostatic tumors is ineffective, so "nipping them in the bud" is a better way to tackle the problem.

Despite the countless considerations that must be weighed when new medications are developed, the single factor that ultimately determines whether a drug is adopted is its toxicity. In chapter 7, we described the drugs used in hormonal therapy, many of which had serious side effects. When a man is dying of prostate cancer, these adverse reactions are acceptable, because the alternative is worse. But when a drug is given to a healthy man for preventive purposes, side effects quickly become unacceptable. This is the main reason hormonal therapy drugs are not being evaluated in prostate cancer prevention, although they would probably be very effective. A drug with any hope of being accepted as a preventive must have limited and mild side effects.

What Potentially Preventive Drugs Are Being Studied?

The drug showing the most promise in preventing prostate cancer is finasteride (Proscar®), which is being used extensively to treat benign prostatic hyperplasia (BPH). Finasteride blocks the chemical 5-α-reductase, which, as we learned in chapter 7, converts testosterone into its more powerful form, DHT. Remember, testosterone and DHT are androgens that stimulate growth of normal as well as cancerous prostate cells. The rationale behind finasteride as a preventive strategy is that males born without 5-α-reductase *never* get prostate cancer. Logically, then, blocking that enzyme should prevent cancer.

Finasteride inhibits 5-α-reductase and depresses blood DHT concentrations to castration levels. Castration is a desired end because men who are castrated before age 40 almost never get prostatic carcinoma. Sexual side effects from finasteride are uncommon, because the chemical castration is incomplete, which means most men can enjoy the benefits of the drug while retaining their potency and sex drive. Because finasteride works only in the prostate gland, side effects are generally rare, mild, and reversible. It may be the ideal preventive!

Unfortunately, things rarely are as simple as they appear. Some research scientists have suggested that finasteride may make matters worse in certain cases. They question whether a decrease in blood DHT necessarily means a decrease in DHT within the prostate. They believe finasteride can *increase* not decrease the concentration of testosterone in the prostate, thus providing fuel for cancer cells to multiply. They are concerned that blocking cancer cells that respond to hormones may favor those that do not, although other researchers do not believe this. At this point, it appears that finasteride assists rather than blocks the development of cancer in a small percentage of men. Who is affected seems to be related to other risk factors like age, race, and family history. Obviously, if and when finasteride is approved for prostate cancer prevention, some men will be advised not to take it. Details should be clearer after the current research studies at the National Cancer Institute (NCI) are completed in the year 2000.

Another group of preventive agents with the potential to make matters worse rather than better is the synthetic retinoid class of vitamin A-like drugs, including the experimental drug 4-HPR. Retinoids inhibit cancer cell growth. But like finasteride, they actually enhance cancer growth in some men. This may be a moot point, because retinoids have too many side effects, like fatigue and impairing one's ability to adapt to low light, ever to allow them to be adopted as a preventive.

An essential chemical reaction that takes place when all human cells, whether normal or cancerous, are stimulated to multiply is conversion of the chemical ornithine to putrescine with the help of the catalyst ornithine decarboxylase (ODC). Putrescine is in a class of chemicals called the polyamines, found in all living things. When more poly-amines are made, more cells multiply, and ODC helps make that happen. Cell multiplication is good when cells are normal, but bad when cells are cancerous. More aggressive cancers have more aggressive ODC, which means more aggressive tumor growth.

Understanding this chemical reaction has led to development of the drug DFMO, which binds to and blocks ODC, thus preventing cancer growth. The prostate has more polyamines than just about any other organ in the body, so DFMO may be a valuable preventive agent. The best thing about DFMO is that it is easy to take orally and has few side effects. There is still research to be done, but scientists are optimistic about its potential to prevent prostatic carcinoma.

Cancer often arises in areas that have been inflamed for long periods. Inflammation of the respiratory tract by cigarette smoke, for example, can cause normal lining cells in the airways to become cancerous. Similar changes can occur when a high-fat, low-fiber diet irritates the lining of the colon. This type of inflammation is mediated by a class of compounds called eicosanoids that are formed from arachidonic acid (AA) with the help of the catalyst PLA2. Many scientists believe eicosanoids give cancer the "green light" to metastasize.

Researchers are beginning to study a potent anti-inflammatory protein called uteroglobin, found in the uterus, respiratory tract, and prostate, which may be effective in blocking the cancer-causing inflammation triggered by the eicosanoids. Uteroglobin blocks PLA2 actions and the release of AA from prostate tumor cells, inhibiting inflammation in the inflammation-prone prostate gland. The net effect of uteroglobin is not that it prevents cancer from forming, but that it keeps prostate cancer cells from spreading beyond their point of origin. Put another way, uteroglobin inhibits the invasiveness not the inception of cancer. This is an exciting discovery whose significance in potentially reducing the number of untreatable prostate tumors is easy to appreciate. Other investigational drugs are currently being evaluated by NCI, but it will be years before their preventive value is known.

What About Diet and Exercise?

There are correlations between diet and exercise and prostate cancer, but few are strong and many are contra-dictory. For example, many researchers have stated that vitamins A and C protect against carcinoma of the prostate. At the same time, others have said that a high in-take of these vitamins increases a man's risk for acquiring the disease. That confusion doesn't help you at all, but it is probably safe to say that a single multivitamin tablet a day is beneficial for most people. Excessive vitamin doses, however, are at the very least wasteful, and quite often harmful.

A stronger association exists between prostate cancer and fat intake. Dietary fat is converted by the body to an-drogens, which, as we know, stimulate growth of cancer cells. Men who eat high-fat diets have a much higher rate of prostate cancer than those who adhere to diets low in fat and rich in yellow and green vegetables. This risk seems to be isolated to animal fats, which are broken down into chemicals that are carcinogenic, or cancer-caus-ing, to prostate cells. Unfortunately, you must have a life-time habit of eating a high-fiber, low-fat diet to benefit from this protective effect. This is one of the reasons why Asians have such a low incidence of prostatic carcinoma when compared to Americans. Switching to this type of diet later in life is not likely to improve your prostate cancer risk, but it is helpful in preventing other problems, such as coronary artery disease and obesity, so it always is a good idea to reduce your intake of saturated fats.

One research study has discovered a correlation between exercise and prostate cancer. Investigators found that men who burned 4000 Calories or more a week, equivalent to about an hour of vigorous exercise a day, had a much lower risk for prostate cancer than men who burned fewer than 1000 Calories a week. The reason was that, as with the dietary fat connection, increased exercise produced lower levels of prostate-stimulating androgens. This is probably the only study of its kind and must therefore be considered carefully. However, low-impact, aerobic-type exercises are a good idea for most people.

Sunshine and vitamin D have a special relationship with each other and with prostate cancer. Experts have known for a long time that vitamin D inhibits growth of cancer cells. Unfortunately, most Americans typically consume only small amounts of this nutrient. Other than fortified milk, there are very few good dietary sources of vitamin D. Fish liver oils are a rich source, an additional reason why Asians, with their fish-concentrated diets, have a low rate of prostate cancer.

Most of the vitamin D we need to live is manufactured in our bodies with the assistance of ultraviolet radiation from the sun. A prohormone in the skin is converted into a previtamin when skin is exposed to sunlight. The previtamin travels to the liver where it is converted into 25-OHD, which travels to the kidney to become vitamin D.

Ultraviolet radiation and vitamin D both protect against prostate cancer. States in the southern half of the U.S., where the sun shines brighter and longer, have lower prostate cancer rates than those in the northern half. Major cities where smog blocks the sun have higher rates than rural areas, where skies are clearer. This may explain why older men and black men have such high incidences of prostatic carcinoma. The melanin in dark skin can block the sun from reaching the prohormone, thus inhibiting production of vitamin D, and older men usually spend more time indoors away from the sun than younger men.

Each of these theories makes sense, but none explains why farmers have such a high incidence of prostate cancer. Because farmers spend so much time outdoors, their ultraviolet exposure should protect them from prostate cancer. But that is not the case as we learned in chapter 2, which stresses the importance of not concentrating on a single risk factor. All relevant information must be taken into account when assessing someone's likelihood for acquiring prostate cancer. Regardless, all this information should give you a good excuse to drink your milk and get outside!

Remember when your mother told you always to eat your brussels sprouts? It turns out she was doing it for good reason. Vegetables like sprouts have been shown to enhance the natural ability of your body cells to resist cancer-causing agents. Not only does the prostate benefit from that effect, but so do other organs. Cauliflower and its relatives accomplish that task by stimulating production of special chemicals like glutathione S-transferase, a catalyst involved in important chemical reactions. Asians tend to eat more broccoli and its relatives than Americans, which adds another item to our list of reasons for the significant difference in prostate cancer rates between the hemispheres.

Recently, a group of scientists discovered a specific mutation in the genetic codes of certain men that impairs their ability to manufacture glutathione S-transferase. This mutation typically occurs late in life and when it does, greatly increases a man's vulnerability to prostate cancer. This is significant not only because it may help identify the cause of prostate cancer, but a test for glutathione S-transferase may eventually be an effective early detection method for prostatic carcinoma.

What's Going on at NCI?

The Prostate Cancer Prevention Trial (PCPT) began October 13, 1993, and will continue until the year 2000. Some 18,000 men are involved in the experiment, which is intended to assess the usefulness of finasteride (Proscar®) in preventing prostate cancer. This is a tough task for four reasons. First, prostate cancer grows very slowly, so test subjects must be followed for a long time to determine whether the drug works. Second, because these men are in their sixties or older, many will die during the course of the study from causes other than prostate cancer. Third, microscopic cancers are extremely common in men in this age group, so it is difficult to find subjects with "clean" prostates. Finally, biopsies must be taken periodically to see whether the drug works, but it is extremely difficult to precisely sample the same area each time. Time will tell what the results of the study will be.

Besides the PCPT, NCI has hundreds of other potentially useful agents on its drawing board. But the consuming public will not see any of them for years. It takes about 12 years of testing for a drug to reach the market.

Chapter 10

What Are the Psychological Considerations of Prostate Cancer?

This may be the most important chapter in this book, so you should share it with your spouse and other members of your immediate family, because it is meant as much for them as for you. If you have just been diagnosed with prostate cancer, this undoubtedly is one of the most significant moments of your life. But it is also significant for those who love you, because they are not only faced with the possibility of losing you, but with a serious disruption of the lifestyle to which they have grown accustomed. If you have friends and family close to you, try not to think your disease affects only you. After all, there are advantages to not having to tackle a serious illness all alone. Pass this chapter on to your wife or loved ones as soon as you read it.

In the previous chapters we discussed life expectancy, length of time without symptoms, length of time to disease progression, and other *quantity* of life concepts relating to prostate cancer. In this chapter, we will address quality of life for men with prostatic carcinoma. Your personal definition of quality of life certainly differs from everybody else's, because we each have unique life experiences, physical attributes, social interactions, and views of the world that influence our individual priorities. Even so, whatever concerns you may have probably have been felt by some other man with prostate cancer.

Why Is Quality of Life Important in Prostate Cancer?

Quality of life is important in every illness. What good is treatment intervention if it only gives you an added year of life filled with unhappiness and discomfort? Quality of life is especially important in prostate cancer because it is such a common disease, and anything that causes pain or psychological distress is bound to affect a lot of men. We already know that treatment methods for advanced stages of prostate cancer are less than 100 percent effective and carry a number of potentially serious side effects. Sometimes, as we discussed in chapter 8, quality of life can be better without treatment.

Odds are when you first found out you had cancer, your immediate reaction was fear. Fear of pain, both from the disease and from treatment, and fear of death are common and normal. Many men describe their initial response to the news as one of helplessness or hopelessness. That was the case with Lee N., who wondered if he would be able to continue his duties as head of the household. He had many new monetary concerns like how he was going to pay for the expensive tests and treatment he'd need. He was also worried that if long-term rehabilitation was necessary, he would be financially unable to miss time from work. Stuck in this scenario, Lee, like many men, was tempted to overlook his condition and ignore the help he needed. Fortunately, his friends and family convinced him how unwise that would be.

Kent L. described his initial reaction as complete disbelief. He could not believe such a thing was happening to him. He walked around in a dreamlike state for weeks. Not until after his surgery was he able to regain his hold on reality.

An ominous diagnosis like cancer disrupts a man's life routine at an age when change is not eagerly embraced. Typically, men with prostate cancer are 60 or older and their wives are also in the latter part of their years. Many of these women have medical problems that require assistance from their husbands, and when these men are suddenly given the extra onus of having to deal with prostate cancer, they often put their own problems on the back burner, because the condition impairs their role as caregiver to their wives. If you are like most men, you probably had one or two pre-existing medical conditions of your own before you were ever diagnosed with prostate cancer. You might have been tempted once or twice to avoid treatment so as not to disturb your usual routine. If so, hopefully you, like Lee N., realize you and your wife will both suffer from such a decision.

Many men react to a diagnosis of prostate cancer with shame and embarrassment. Genital organs, urinary function, and sexual performance are not topics men feel comfortable discussing freely, but these elements compose a major part of society's definition of masculinity. The potential for any or all of them to be adversely affected by prostate cancer or its treatment can deal a tremendous blow to the male ego, one of the reasons the disease was not discussed openly by the general population until recently. Many years ago, women with breast cancer had similar problems gaining public recognition, but now they are enjoying the fruits of their demands for attention. Funds for breast cancer research outnumber prostate cancer research by 8 to 1. But advances are being made rapidly and hardly a day goes by now without a prostate cancer reference appearing in the media.

Psychological, physical, and lifestyle concerns all contribute to the cumbersome excess baggage that accompanies diagnosis of prostate cancer. Such a burden is enough to exhaust even the strongest man. Fatigue is one of the most common complaints of men with prostate cancer. The disease itself, treatment side effects, and the increased need to tend to personal and financial matters can sap a man of every ounce of energy. Despite their fatigue, many men with prostate cancer have trouble getting a good night's rest. Thoughts race through their heads about all the new changes and disruptions in their lives, which makes falling asleep difficult. This explains why men with prostate cancer frequently develop significant depression. This depression can be even more severe if you have undergone surgery or radiation therapy in the hope of being cured, only to find the treatment was unsuccessful. Depression is real, common, and can be treated. But first, you have to make your feelings known to those around you.

If you have prostate cancer, you can probably identify with any or all of the psychological aspects we have discussed. Hopefully, you will recognize you are not alone in the way you feel and you must not allow fear, anger, sadness, or embarrassment to prevent you from doing what is best for you. Remember, there are others who care whether you live or die.

What Is My Wife's Role in All of This?

While men usually have trouble dealing with intimate physical problems, women are far less inhibited. Men frequently are embarrassed when they must discuss genital and rectal examinations, while women, thanks to their regular visits to the gynecologist's office, are quite familiar with these procedures. Women are generally more verbal than men and more likely to establish necessary lines of communication. If you are a man who has just been diagnosed with prostate cancer, consider yourself fortunate if you have a woman by your side, because she is likelier than you are to ask the questions you need to have answered.

This female sensitivity comes at a price. It is common for a wife to be affected more profoundly by her husband's diagnosis of prostate cancer than he is. Typically, men are raised with traditional ideas of masculinity and usually are taught to grin and bear it in the face of adversity. On the other hand, women have no such defense mechanism built in and are usually more vulnerable in crises. While women may be more willing to discuss openly their own health issues, many become uncomfortable when the conversation turns to male health problems.

The effect of your prostate cancer on your spouse may go beyond mere embarrassment or fear. Prostate cancer often strikes men already weakened by age or other medical problems and it can rob them of their last shred of ability to care for themselves or others. When that happens, wives must assume the roles of provider and caregiver. Driving to doctor's appointments, shopping, cooking, cleaning, administering medications, and managing the budget must be taken over by the wife, leaving her little or no time for her own social or recreational activities. That is a tremendous load for these women and it worsens as their husbands grow older and sicker. Mildred P. had to care for her husband, Vincent, after advanced prostate cancer left him bedridden. After months of setting aside her own needs, she began to feel resentment, anger, fatigue, and even depression. Privately, she wished for an end to her husband's terminal condition, not so much to end his suffering, but hers. Even in his debilitated state, Vincent detected these signals from his wife. Mildred felt deeply ashamed of what she considered her evil, selfish feelings. Not until she saw a counselor did she learn that having those feelings was an honest human reaction to extraordinary circumstances.

Should I Discuss These Issues with My Doctor?

Yes, but you will probably have to be the one who raises the subject. Your doctor cares about your psychological well being, but he usually is too immersed in quantity of life matters like diagnosing, staging, and treating your cancer to place quality of life issues at the top of his agenda. Your doctor may have killing the cancer on his mind, but you obviously have additional concerns. You have your own values, beliefs, preferences, and goals that must be taken into account when you plan a strategy for treating your disease. Your doctor cannot read your mind, so it is up to you to lay your cards before him.

In a perfect world, all doctors would ask about your quality of life, but since it is not, pretend your doctor *did* ask you and answer him. Tell him if you have had any problems with normal daily activities like cleaning, dressing, eating, and using the bathroom. Tell him if you have been able to stay active or if you have had problems walking, climbing, bending, or lifting. Tell him about your urinary habits and if you have noticed any significant changes. Tell him about your overall sense of well-being and your energy level. Tell him about psychological concerns like tension, irritability, loneliness, or depression.

This list is far from complete; everything is fair game. You must develop the mind set that it is your body and your life at stake, so you will call the shots.

How Do I Get Help with My Psychological Concerns?

Social workers are an excellent source of psychological and social support when a serious illness upsets your life and those you love. If you are selecting a prostate cancer therapy, a social worker can help you balance all the physical, mental, social, religious, and financial issues involved in making an informed decision. If you are worried about how you will pay for the tests and treatment you will undergo, a social worker can help you deal with insurance carriers and devise a payment strategy. If you wonder how you will get to and from the hospital or radiation suite, a social worker can arrange transportation. If you are unsure where you will stay when you are released from the hospital, a social worker can make arrangements. If care by a visiting nurse is required after you leave the hospital, a social worker can organize this as well.

Social workers provide a convenient option for navigating through the complex bureaucracy of our health care system. Many social workers specialize as doctors do. A urologic social worker understands the special needs of urologic patients, including those who just underwent radical prostatectomies. Similarly, you may encounter an oncologic social worker if you are receiving radiation therapy. Their specialization is good for you because it means you are dealing with somebody who knows about and understands your situation.

Psychiatrists and psychologists can also counsel you. The best way to reach one is with a recommendation from someone you trust, like a friend, family member, or your doctor. Friends and family are good sources of psychological support themselves and should be your first thought when you need someone to talk to. However, you'll probably find the most comfort and sympathy from men who have had prostate cancer themselves. Almost every community in the U.S. has a support group for men with prostate cancer. Ask your doctor for the name and address of a group near you or contact the consumer resource organizations listed in the appendix. All the feelings you are having because of your cancer are normal. Help is just around the corner.

Chapter 11

What Is Benign Prostatic Hyperplasia (BPH)?

We are finished discussing prostate cancer, so let's shift gears and talk about benign prostatic hyperplasia (BPH), a prostate problem less serious from a survival standpoint, equally important from a quality of life perspective, and far more important in terms of the number of men affected. You can understand BPH simply by analyzing its name. Benign is the opposite of malignant. Unlike carcinoma of the prostate, BPH does not metastasize beyond the prostate, so it is less dangerous than cancer. Hyperplasia is an excessive proliferation of normal cells, unlike cancer, where cells are abnormal. Therefore, benign prostatic hyperplasia means a nonmalignant, excessive growth of prostate cells. This may not sound like such a terrible condition, until you recall that the urethra, the tube carrying urine from the bladder to the outside world, runs through the prostate. As BPH develops and grows, the urethra is gradually pinched off, leading to a host of uncomfortable and distressing symptoms.

How Common Is BPH?

Your prostate grows throughout your life, starting very small when you are a child and reaching about 20 grams (¾ ounce) by the time you are 30. That weight remains steady for the next 20 or so years, then it begins to grow again, reaching 35 grams by age 80. Just by living to an advanced age, you will experience a certain amount of prostate growth, but BPH and growth are not necessarily related.

BPH is the most common benign tumor in men. If you are over 50, you have more than a 50 percent chance of having BPH right now. If you live to be 80 to 85, your odds of getting BPH approach 90 percent. Merely having BPH does not require treating it. Only about half the men who have BPH ever have symptoms calling for treatment. If you are a man and live to be 80, you have a 20–30 percent chance of developing BPH requiring treatment.

Still, 20–30 percent of all men is a large number. Therefore, it is really no surprise that transurethral resection of the prostate (TURP), the most popular surgical treatment for BPH, is the second most common operation performed on American men in their sixties or older (cataract extraction is first). Almost 400,000 TURPs are performed each year in the U.S. Add another 15,000 to 40,000 standard open prostatectomies and you've got a lot of operations to treat a benign disease. A typical urologist in the U.S. devotes about 30–40 percent of his practice to BPH, a big problem that affects many men.

Are Some Men More Likely than Others to Get BPH?

To be at risk for BPH you need only be old and male. Some other factors *can* play a role. As with prostate cancer, Asians have a lower incidence of BPH than Americans; Europeans have a higher incidence. Unlike prostate cancer, blacks and whites have an equivalent risk to acquire BPH, although blacks tend to develop symptoms earlier.

A curious relationship exists between BPH and cigarette smoking. Smokers tend to have a *decreased* likelihood of developing BPH. This same protection seems to exist among men who have the liver disease cirrhosis. Men with cirrhosis have a lower incidence of BPH than men with healthy livers, and doctors think it may be because they have higher concentrations of circulating female hormones. Whatever the reason may be, you might be tempted to take that as an invitation to smoke and drink your way out of BPH. If so, you would be trading a single benign disease for two far more serious ones.

Finally, the question everyone asks is whether BPH increases your chance of getting prostate cancer. Unfortunately, research has not been able to resolve this issue. Some studies show increased risk, some show none, and others show a decreased risk. The best way to summarize the data would be to say that no strong relationship between BPH and cancer has yet to be proved. However, it is clear that the same things that put you at risk for BPH—being old and male—also put you at risk for cancer. BPH and cancer also frequently coexist, which is why your doctor carefully examines any tissue removed during an operation for BPH.

What Changes to the Prostate and Bladder Occur in BPH?

In chapter 1, we learned BPH occurs in the periurethral and transition zones of the prostate, the area of tissue that surrounds the urethra as it passes through the gland. The growth begins within the muscular and fibrous cells of the prostate, later expanding to include the fluid-secreting glandular cells. Part of the BPH tissue exists in the form of discrete nodules, another part is more diffuse. As the BPH tissue in the transition and periurethral zones grows, the expanding mass pushes against the surrounding tissue in the central and peripheral zones, which can only be moved so far until it compresses against the outer capsule. BPH growth persists even after there is no more room within the prostate, and that is when the increased pressure begins to squeeze the urethra closed and cause symptoms of urinary obstruction. Other factors, such as muscle fibers surrounding the urethra that are irritated into contracting by the BPH process, compound the obstruction.

Because BPH occurs in the inner part of the prostate immediately surrounding the urethra, the size of the gland has little or no bearing on whether symptoms will ever develop. A small prostate can be severely obstructed; a large prostate can be completely unobstructed.

There is still no satisfactory explanation for BPH. Male hormones seem to play a role, but no one knows whether they stimulate BPH or provide a supportive environment for it. Prostate cancer, BPH, and normal prostate cells all require DHT and other androgens for growth and survival. Castration improves BPH symptoms by removing the supply of DHT in much the same way it does during metastatic cancer treatment. That is the rationale behind finasteride (Proscar®), the most common form of medical treatment for BPH. Other chemicals, called growth factors, are thought to play a role in initiating BPH. Another explanation for BPH could be that cell multiplication exceeds cell death once men reach a certain age. Finally, some researchers have proposed that a lifetime of minor injuries from urinating to ejaculating to getting infections results in triggering BPH as a healing response.

Whatever its cause, BPH can take its toll on the bladder and the rest of the urinary tract. As the tumor encroaches on the urethra, bladder drainage is restricted causing the bladder muscle, the detrusor, to contract with greater force to expel urine. This works for a while and the detrusor becomes thicker and stronger to compensate for its increased effort. These changes persist even after definitive surgical treatment, which explains why some men continue to have urinary symptoms as many as 12 months after a TURP. Eventually, the detrusor loses its ability to force urine through a progressively narrowing urethra. Then the bladder can no longer empty completely and that's when most symptoms begin. If the situation continues, pressure within the bladder continues to increase and not only during voiding. This is dangerous, because the pressure is transmitted back through the urinary tract into the kidneys, where permanent and life-threatening damage can take place. Fortunately, this is rare, because most men are driven by their symptoms to seek medical attention long before serious complications occur.

What Are the Symptoms of BPH?

Prostatism is often used to refer to the collection of symptoms caused by BPH. BPH symptoms can be divided into two categories—obstructive symptoms, related directly to the squeezing effect of BPH on the urethra, and irritative symptoms, manifestations of the instability of the detrusor muscle, a consequence of the obstruction. Some men with BPH are obstructed but have no symptoms; this is silent prostatism.

Obstructive symptoms include hesitancy, weak stream, intermittency, incomplete emptying, and terminal dribbling. Hesitancy is an increase in the period between when you initiate urination by relaxing your urethral sphincter and when the urine stream actually begins. In men without BPH, this interval should only be a few seconds, but a lack of privacy during urination can also cause hesitancy of the "shy kidney" type. You may recognize a *weak* stream not only by its being less forceful, but also by its being thinner than usual. Most men are aware of what is normal for them. Intermittency is an interruption of the urinary stream in the middle of voiding. Incomplete voiding is a desire to urinate immediately after you already have done so. Left untreated, that can lead to urinary tract infections or urinary retention, which we'll discuss later. Terminal dribbling is a low-level flow for several seconds at the end of urination, a sign the detrusor muscle can no longer maintain a full-force stream.

Irritative symptoms include frequency, nocturia, urgency, urge incontinence, dysuria, hematuria, enuresis, urinary tract infection, and urinary retention. Frequency refers to abnormally frequent trips to the toilet, which usually means more than 7 times a day or fewer than 3 hours between visits. Obviously, a lot depends upon your fluid intake, whether you've taken diuretics, and other factors. Being awakened in the middle of the night by the urge to void is nocturia, which is not the same as awakening first, then noticing the urge. Older men typically excrete most of their urine at night, so a trip to the bathroom at a late hour is not necessarily abnormal. Urgency is an overwhelming need to urinate, often accompanied by the sensation that leakage, or urge incontinence, will occur if the need isn't satisfied. Dysuria is painful urination, often described as a feeling of "passing broken glass." A similar symptom is strangury, urethral pain at the end of voiding. Both dysuria and strangury are characteristic of urinary tract infections, which are common in men who have symptomatic BPH, but rare in men who don't. This probably is due to several factors, including decreased "washing" force of the urinary stream, stagnant urine remaining in the bladder after voiding, and diminished defense mechanisms in the bladder. Hematuria, or blood in the urine, and enuresis, or bedwetting, are uncommon symptoms of BPH.

About 20 percent of men with obstruction from BPH suffer acute retention, the sudden inability to urinate. Men with BPH often adapt to the symptoms we've listed so far, but few can avoid medical attention once acute retention develops. Quickly and easily relieved by passing a catheter into the bladder, acute retention usually signals the need for definitive treatment of underlying BPH. Chronic retention is a more gradual process and is not harmful as long as pressure within the bladder is low and the retained urine is uninfected. If the pressure rises, however, it can be transmitted backward to the kidneys and lead to kidney failure, uremia, and death. Fortunately, this is a rare occurrence.

None of these symptoms are specific for BPH. Any can be caused by a number of other conditions. Obstructive symptoms can be caused by urethral strictures, bladder neck contractures, bladder stones, or carcinoma of the prostate or bladder. Irritative symptoms can be caused by detrusor muscle instability, urinary tract infections, prostate inflammation, or diabetes.

BPH symptoms can be exacerbated by some of the medications you might be taking for other conditions. Stimulants, such as those in certain asthma medications and sinus decongestants, can narrow the urethra even more. Other drugs, such as many of the antispasm medications, can diminish the bladder's ability to expel urine. Diuretics and alcoholic beverages can also make matters worse, which is why it's important to give your doctor a complete list of all of your medications (including over-the-counter drugs). Stopping an offending medication may be all you need to do to correct your symptoms.

There are many symptoms that can be caused by BPH, and each man can suffer from a unique combination of any or all. This can make it difficult for a urologist to decide which symptoms are more pressing and when medical intervention is indicated. To standardize symptom evaluation from one BPH case to another, the American Urological Association (AUA) has compiled a symptom index (Table 11.1) so your doctor can assign a number to your individual collection of symptoms. A score between 0 and 7 is considered mild, 8 to 19 moderate, and 20 to 35 severe. The higher your score, the likelier it is that you need treatment.

How Is BPH Diagnosed?

Undoubtedly, the most important part of the diagnostic workup for BPH is the history of symptoms you describe to your doctor. Your doctor may even ask you to keep a diary of your urinary habits, so he can assess how frequently and with what severity certain symptoms occur. The history includes other medical problems, especially neurological conditions like Parkinson's disease and stroke, which can cause urinary obstruction all by themselves. The existence of other medical conditions is also important in determining your fitness for surgery.

A complete physical examination is essential to reaching a diagnosis. Special attention is paid to the digital rectal exam and to the neurological exam. Laboratory tests include a urinalysis to rule out blood or infection in the urine and a blood creatinine level to assess kidney function. On the basis of a history, physical exam, lab tests,

---

Table 11.1
The American Urological Association Symptom Index

---

1. Over the past month, how often have you had a sensation of not emptying your bladder completely after you finished urinating?
2. Over the past month, how often have you had to urinate again less than 2 hours after you finished urinating?
3. Over the past month, how often have you found you stopped and started again several times when you urinated?
4. Over the past month, how often have you found it difficult to postpone urination?
5. Over the past month, how often have you had a weak urinary stream?
6. Over the past month, how often have you had to push or strain to begin urination?
7. Over the past month, how many times did you most typically get up to urinate from the time you went to bed at night until the time you got up in the morning?

For each question, give a score of 0 for "not at all," 1 for "less than 1-in-5 times," 2 for "less than half the time," 3 for "about half the time," 4 for "more than half the time," and 5 for "almost always." For question 7, add the appropriate number of times.

and AUA symptom index, your urologist can usually diagnose BPH with a high degree of confidence.

Other more sophisticated tests are available when the diagnosis is uncertain. Uroflowmetry is an inexpensive, painless test that can provide useful information. It involves is drinking lots of fluids until you're ready to urinate, then voiding into the machine, which measures the flow rate of your stream. A flow rate less than 10 milliliters (about ⅓ fl. oz.) per second suggests urinary obstruction. Remember, your doctor cannot attribute an obstruction to BPH with 100 percent certainty purely on the basis of uroflowmetry. Other conditions, such as urethral strictures, can also cause obstruction.

When more information is needed, pressure-flow studies can be performed, although they are seldom used. This test measures not only your urinary flow, but the actual pressures within your bladder and urethra. A special catheter with pressure sensors is inserted into your urethra and advanced into your bladder. Pressure readings are taken and compared with the normal range, which is about 20–35 centimeters of water. A man with urinary obstruction can have a bladder pressure of 40–80 cm H_2O or more. Your bladder is then filled with an x-ray contrast solution and your doctor watches an x-ray screen and videotape monitor while you urinate. Pressure-flow studies are far more specific than uroflowmetry for distinguishing BPH from bladder dysfunction.

Another diagnostic technique used occasionally in BPH workups is post-void residual measurement, which checks the amount of urine in your bladder after voiding. It can be performed using a catheter or an ultrasound device. Cystoscopy is not used routinely in diagnosing BPH, but can be used to measure the size and shape of the prostate when surgery has already been planned. Intravenous pyelography (IVP) is reserved for complicated situations involving stones, blood, infection, or kidney failure.

Should My BPH Be Treated?

In some cases, the answer is an unequivocal yes. Kidney failure from urinary obstruction, recurrent urinary tract infections, large volumes of blood in the urine, bladder stones, and acute retention that fails to respond to catheterization are all scenarios that require definitive treatment, usually surgical. In other cases, provided your AUA symptom index is less than 7, the answer is almost certainly no. The rest of the men with BPH must decide among surgery, medication, or "watching-and-waiting." The option you choose depends on how badly your symptoms disrupt your lifestyle. In the next chapter you'll learn about the various treatment methods, so that you can make an informed decision.

Chapter 12

How Is BPH Treated?

The therapeutic options for BPH are far less contro-versial than those for prostate cancer. In most BPH cases, it's fairly clear who needs treatment and who doesn't. Once the decision to treat has been made, usually it is not difficult to determine whether surgical or medical therapy should be employed. BPH is not a life-threatening illness, except in those rare cases that cause kidney failure, so therapy is instituted solely to relieve symptoms. Mild symptoms, those that correspond to a score of 7 or less on the AUA index we learned about in the last chapter, are usually best handled with a "watching-and-waiting" strat-egy. That includes limiting nighttime fluid intake, avoid-ing nasal decongestant drugs, and paying regular visits to your doctor. Symptoms worse than mild open up the menu of treatment possibilities.

Surgical procedures for BPH range from open prostatec-tomy to transurethral resection of the prostate (TURP) to transurethral incision of the prostate (TUIP). Balloon di-latation is also being used by some urologists, although it is still officially classified as experimental. Medications for BPH include α_1-blockers like terazosin (Hytrin®) and 5-α-reductase inhibitors like finasteride (Proscar®). Newer treatment methods currently under investigation run the gamut from laser prostatectomy to microwave thermal therapy to urethral stents. The objective of scientists developing these new techniques is to find ways to treat BPH that are less involved and, therefore, safer than surgery.

Obviously, you have many therapy choices if you have BPH, but the options vary in their degree of success in relieving symptoms. The surgical procedures as a group are significantly better in improving urinary flow than the medical alternatives. Medication is superior to watching-and-waiting in terms of symptomatic relief. Why then would anyone deliberately choose a less effective means of therapy? We'll answer this question by describing each type of treatment separately.

What Types of BPH Surgery Are There?

The standard surgical procedure for BPH is transurethral resection of the prostate (TURP), which, as its name implies, is performed through the urethra rather than through a skin incision. A long, thin instrument called a resectoscope is inserted into the urethra and advanced until the urologist can see the BPH tissue. He then cuts away the excess tissue bit by bit using an electrical loop at the end of the resectoscope. The advantage of TURP is that it provides samples of prostatic tissue that can be sent to the laboratory to check for cancer. After the operation, a moderate amount of bleeding remains, so a Foley catheter is left in your urethra through which bladder irrigation can be done.

Transurethral incision of the prostate (TUIP) deserves to be used a lot more than it is at present. Similar to TURP, instead of removing all of the BPH tissue, TUIP involves cutting through it to loosen the obstruction to urinary flow. An electric knife is used to make two deep incisions beginning just inside the bladder and extending down into the prostatic urethra. TUIP is faster, safer, and cheaper than TURP, so it is a good option for men like Barry L., whose coronary artery disease and diabetes made him too much of an operative risk for the more complex TURP. Unfortunately, TUIP only works well on small prostates.

We learned about open prostatectomy in chapter 5. This can be performed through a retropubic approach, involving a below-the-navel incision and opening the prostate to reach the BPH tissue, or through a suprapubic approach, entailing the same incision and reaching the prostate by opening the bladder. TURP and TUIP have all but replaced open prostatectomy as a form of treatment for BPH, but the open procedure still is used for very large prostates. The suprapubic approach, in particular, is good when bladder stones are present.

In most instances, symptomatic BPH is a disease best treated with surgery—the standard against which all other treatment methods are measured. In some situations such as unresponsive acute urinary retention, kidney failure due to BPH, severe bloody urine, frequent urinary tract infections, and bladder stones, surgery is the *only* acceptable option. It is clearly the best choice when the urinary obstruction severely compromises the urinary flow rate.

Any medical or surgical intervention carries a number of potential side effects and BPH surgery is no exception. In most cases, TURP, TUIP, and open prostatectomy eliminate the bladder neck's ability to close during ejaculation, which means during ejaculation semen flows backward into the bladder instead of forward into the urethra. This is retrograde ejaculation and it occurs in 70–75 percent of TURPs and open prostatectomies, but only in about 25 percent of TUIPs. Retrograde ejaculation is not dangerous and you can enjoy normal sexual relations despite it, but conceiving children is not possible because the sperm travel in the wrong direction. Bob G. continued to have an active sex life after his TURP, despite retrograde ejaculation. He described the feeling as being different, but not uncomfortable or bothersome.

Impotence and incontinence are two rare but genuine risks of BPH surgery. Open prostatectomy carries a 12–13 percent chance of impotence, while TURP and TUIP are a little better at 7–9 percent. Incontinence occurs far less frequently, with 1½–2 percent of men losing bladder control only at times of stress, such as when lifting or coughing, and fewer than 1 percent being incontinent all of the time. Obviously these figures are rough estimates; the numbers vary widely depending on the data source.

TURP, TUIP, and open prostatectomy also have the same general risks that any other operation under anesthesia would have. These include infection, fever, bleeding, and wound complications. A unique collection of side effects called the TURP syndrome, which includes mental confusion, nausea and vomiting, high blood pressure, slow heart rate, and vision changes, follows a small number of TURPs and occurs when the irrigation fluid used during the procedure is inadvertently absorbed into the bloodstream. Finally, BPH surgery also carries a 1–3 percent risk of narrowing the urethra and bladder neck by scar tissue.

Death is a possibility with any major operation. Few men die during a TURP, TUIP, or open prostatectomy, but some die shortly afterward from complications, such as heart attack or stroke. It would make sense that open prostatectomy, the most complicated of the procedures, would have the highest mortality rate and TUIP, the simplest, would have the lowest rate, with TURP somewhere in the middle; that is not the case. For some reason the experts have yet to figure out, TURP has a slighly higher mortality rate than open prostatectomy. Most doctors believe it has something to do with the fact that men selected for open prostatectomy usually are in better physical shape than those who undergo TURP. In any case, the risk of death from *any* of these procedures is very small and should not frighten you away from getting necessary treatment.

TURP, TUIP, and open prostatectomy are not equal in their effectiveness in correcting BPH symptoms. In general, open prostatectomy has a higher success rate than TURP, which has a higher success rate than TUIP. The choice among the three depends on the size and shape of your individual prostate gland, so your urologist must ultimately make the decision. Any of the surgical procedures is far more effective than the best of the medical options. The benefits don't always last forever, though. Some 15–20 percent of men who have a TURP must undergo another within 6–8 years, because of scar tissue or new BPH growth.

Finally, you would expect open prostatectomy to be the most expensive of the procedures and to involve the longest hospital stay, and it is and does. If you have an open prostatectomy, you can expect to be hospitalized for 5–10 days. TURP and TUIP allow shorter stays, at 3–4 days and 1–2 days, respectively.

What Types of Medication Are Used for BPH?

The medications available today are less effective than surgery for treating BPH. However, they do have their place. Medical treatment is ideal for someone who is not medically fit to undergo surgery or for someone like Harry

K., who just couldn't stomach the idea of someone operating on his genital area. Medication is also appropriate for symptoms too severe for watching-and-waiting, but not severe enough to warrant surgery. Two drawbacks of medical therapy are that it does not provide a tissue sample that can be checked for cancer, so you must continue with your annual rectal exams and PSA tests, and it must be taken for the duration of your life to prevent a relapse of symptoms.

The first class of medications used for BPH are the α_1-blockers, which include terazosin (Hytrin®), prazosin (Minipress®), and doxazosin (Cardura®). All three are used for high blood pressure and work by relaxing the smooth muscle in the walls of blood vessels. Similarly, much of the obstruction that is present in BPH is caused by contraction of smooth muscle in the walls of the urethra. Giving an α-blocker breaks this grip and restores the flow of urine from the bladder. Today, only terazosin is approved by the FDA for use in BPH. However, clinical judgment allows your doctor to use any of the three.

Doses of α-blockers used in BPH are smaller than for high blood pressure, so their effects on your blood pressure are usually inconsequential. The typical dose is given at bedtime and increased gradually over several weeks to minimize side effects. The most common adverse reactions are tiredness, weakness, headaches, dizziness, and nasal congestion. More severe reactions include a drop in blood pressure when standing, severe dizziness, and fainting. Retrograde ejaculation occurs about 6 percent of the time.

In chapter 9, we learned about finasteride (Proscar®), the 5-α-reductase inhibitor that causes partial castration by stopping DHT production, the active form of testosterone. By cutting off the male hormone fuel to the BPH tissue, finasteride causes a reduction in prostate size and an increase in the urine flow rate. As a result of its hormonal effects, a small number of men taking this drug have problems with impotence and lack of sexual desire. Overall, though, its safety profile is very good. Finasteride takes longer to begin working than an α-blocker, so the latter is often used as a supplement until Proscar® reaches its full effects.

Several factors can help determine which medication should be selected. If a biopsy is available, it can be examined for glandular and muscular composition. BPH that is mostly muscle is best treated with terazosin, because the drug targets this tissue specifically. BPH that is mostly glandular is more susceptible to the hormonal manipulations of finasteride. Sam R. was already taking a medication for blood pressure when he was diagnosed with BPH, so his doctor, wishing not to compound the drug's effects by adding terazosin, prescribed finasteride instead. Both finasteride and terazosin have equivalent success rates at around 70 percent or so.

What Is Balloon Dilatation?

Balloon dilatation is a new therapeutic technique that physically disrupts BPH-induced urinary obstruction without requiring surgery. It involves placing a special catheter into the prostatic urethra and inflating a balloon at the end of the catheter. The balloon pushes against the obstructing tissue and forces open a channel through which urine can exit the bladder. The procedure can usually be done on an outpatient basis under local anesthesia.

Balloon dilatation is not for everyone, especially men with very large prostates. It works well for men with smaller glands or for those who are medically unfit to undergo a prostatectomy. The main problem with balloon treatment is its high failure rate. As many as half the men who have it done suffer a return of symptoms within a year; those who make it through the first year usually do well after that. Some American urologists are already starting to use the balloon technique, even though it is considered an experimental treatment. The future of balloon therapy appears bleak, however, because of its unacceptable failure rate.

What Other New Treatments Are There for BPH?

Lasers are the wave of the future in all types of surgery and urology is no exception. In the treatment of BPH, the neodymium yttrium aluminum garnet (YAG) laser is being used to destroy unwanted tissue. A laser probe is inserted through the urethra under the guidance of ultrasound or cystoscopy and a sideways-firing beam vaporizes the obstructing tumor. The laser generates very high temperatures, so general anesthesia and an overnight hospital stay are required. As with balloon dilatation, some urologists have incorporated the laser into their practice despite its experimental status. It is clear, however, that laser's popularity will grow exponentially over the next several years.

We discussed hyperthermia therapy in chapter 6. This is the experimental treatment where a microwave probe is placed in the rectum or urethra and the prostate is heated in order to kill cancer cells. The same principal is being investigated in the treatment of BPH. The only difference between cancer and BPH cells is that the latter require higher temperatures before they are destroyed. Therefore, hyperthermia, involving temperatures below 45°C (113°F) has evolved into thermal therapy, where temperatures exceed 45°C. Thermal therapy requires up to 10 individual treatments, all done on an outpatient basis. One day it will be a reasonable option for men who are too ill to undergo surgery.

The last form of BPH treatment currently under investigation is the urethral stent. This is simply a flexible, tube-shaped metal coil or mesh that is inserted into the prostatic urethra as a means of holding it open. There are two kinds of stents. Temporary stents are a simple, inexpensive form of urinary retention relief for men too old or too sick for surgery. As their name implies, they occasionally need to be replaced if they become clogged or infected. Permanent stents are more expensive, but last longer because their inner surface acquires a coating of new cells, which essentially makes the stent part of the urethra.

The present and future treatment options for BPH are myriad, ranging from watching-and-waiting to open prostatectomy, from TURP to TUIP, from α-blockers to 5-α-reductase inhibitors, from balloons to stents, and from lasers to thermal therapy. With so many choices, there is bound to be something for all prostates, big and small, and for all men, sick and healthy. Therefore, there is no reason why you should have to live with the uncomfortable symptoms of BPH.

APPENDIX:
Where Can I Get More Information?

Organizations

American Cancer Society
1599 Clifton Rd.
Atlanta, GA 30329
(800) ACS-2345
Consumer information and assistance

American Foundation for Urologic Disease
300 West Pratt St., Ste. 401
Baltimore, MD 21201
(800) 242-2383
Consumer information and sponsor of US-TOO

National Cancer Institute
The National Institutes of Health
Bethesda, MD 20892
(800) 4-CANCER
Consumer information and status of ongoing clinical trials

Patient Advocates for Advanced Cancer Treatments (PAACT)
1143 Parmalee NW
Grand Rapids, MI 49504
(616) 453-1477
Information on advanced cancer treatments

Prostate Cancer Education Council
1180 Avenue of the Americas
New York, NY 10036
(212) 221-3300
Consumer information

US-TOO
c/o American Foundation for Urologic Disease
300 West Pratt St., Ste. 401
Baltimore, MD 21201
(800) 82-US-TOO
Prostate cancer support group.

Brochures

"The ABC's of BPH." Abbott Laboratories; P.O. Box 025590; Miami, FL 33102-9717; (800) 444-1117.

"About Prostatectomy (for Benign Prostatic Hyperplasia)." American College of Surgeons; 55 East Erie St.; Chicago, IL 60611.

"Before, During, and After Your Radical Prostatectomy." American Foundation for Urologic Disease.

"Cancer Communication: Prostate Cancer Report." PAACT.

"Cancer Facts for Men." American Cancer Society.

"Enlarged Prostate: BPH and Other Male Urinary Problems." American Foundation for Urologic Disease.

"Facts on Prostate Cancer." American Cancer Society.

"For Men Only: What You Should Know About Prostate Cancer." American Cancer Society.

"For Women Who Care: Information on Prostate Disease to Share with the Men in Your Life." American Foundation for Urologic Disease.

"Prostate Cancer: Some Good News Men Can Live With." Prostate Cancer Education Council.

"Prostate Cancer: Vital Information for Men Over 40." American Foundation for Urologic Disease.

"Prostate Cancer: What Every Man Over 40 Should Know." American Foundation for Urologic Disease.

"Prostate Cancer: What It Is and How It Is Treated." Zeneca Pharmaceuticals Group; Professional Services; 1800 Concord Pike; Wilmington, DE 19897.

"Prostate Enlargement: Benign Prostatic Hyperplasia." National Kidney and Urologic Diseases Information Clearinghouse; Box NKUDIC; Bethesda, MD 20892.

"Questions and Answers About Zoladex® and Prostate Cancer Treatment." Zeneca Pharmaceuticals.

"Questions and Answers on Lupron Depot®." TAP Pharmaceuticals, Inc.; 2355 Waukegan Rd.; Deerfield, IL 60015.

"Radiation Therapy and You." National Cancer Institute.

"Sexuality and Cancer: For the Man Who Has Cancer and His Partner." American Cancer Society.

"Taking Time: Support for People with Cancer and the People Who Care About Them." National Cancer Institute.

"Treating Your Enlarged Prostate: Patient Guide." AHCPR Publications Clearinghouse; P.O. Box 8547; Silver Spring, MD 20907; (800) 358-9295.

"What You Need to Know About Prostate Cancer." National Cancer Institute.

"When Cancer Recurs: Meeting the Challenge Again." National Cancer Institute.

GLOSSARY

5-α-reductase: Enzyme responsible for converting testosterone into its active form, DHT.

5-α-reductase inhibitor: Class of drug used in treatment of BPH.

acid phosphatase: Enzyme produced by the prostate and whose blood level was instrumental in diagnosis of prostate disease until discovery of prostate-specific antigen (PSA).

acinus (pl. acini): Individual fluid-producing glandular unit of the prostate.

acute urinary retention: Sudden inability to urinate.

adenocarcinoma: Malignant neoplasm arising in the glandular tissue of an organ. Type of cancer seen most often in the prostate.

adjuvant therapy: Any treatment given supplementally to the primary therapy.

adrenal: Triangular-shaped gland resting atop the kidney. Responsible for secreting a number of hormones, including androgens.

adrenocorticotropic hormone (ACTH): Chemical produced by the pituitary gland and which stimulates adrenal gland into secreting its hormones.

age-specific reference ranges: Normal values of laboratory studies adjusted for variances that occur with advancing age.

α_1-**blocker**: Class of antihypertensive drug used to relax the obstruction that occurs in BPH.

ampulla: Terminal, widened portion of vas deferens.

androgens: Hormones secreted by the testes and adrenals and which are responsible for male traits: body hair, deep voice, and sperm production.

aneuploid: Having abnormal number of chromosomes.

atypical adenomatous hyperplasia (AAH): Precancerous condition of the prostate characterized by small, round, uniform, tightly packed glandular units (acini) with tiny excretory ducts branching off of normal, pre-existing ducts.

balloon dilatation: Experimental form of treatment for BPH in which a catheter with a balloon at one end is inserted through the urethra and inflated to force open the obstruction.

benign: Not tending toward metastasis.

benign prostatic hyperplasia (BPH): Nonmalignant excessive growth of prostate cells.

biopsy: Sample of tissue used for diagnostic purposes.

bone scintigraphy: (Also bone scan). Nuclear medicine study used to locate areas of increased bone buildup and degradation.

brachytherapy: (Also interstitial implants). Radiation therapy in which radioactive source is inserted into the prostate itself.

bulbourethral gland: (Also Cowper's gland). One of two male accessory glands producing ingredients for semen.

calculus (pl. calculi): (Also a stone). Prostatic concretion that has hardened from calcium deposit.

cancer: Uncontrolled proliferation of abnormal cells that if left untreated takes control of an entire organ or even the entire body. Malignant neoplasm.

capsule: Thick layer of fibrous tissue encasing the prostate.

carcinogenesis: Production or origin of cancer.

carcinoma: Cancer arising in visceral organs like the lung, breast, colon, and prostate.

carcinoma in situ: Last grade of a premalignant condition such as PIN or AAH before it crosses the basal cell layer and becomes invasive cancer.

central zone: Region of the prostate where ejaculatory ducts empty into urethra and where prostate cancer is least often found.

chronic urinary retention: Gradually evolving inability to urinate.

colliculus seminalis: (See verumontanum).

collimators: Metal shields used to protect nontarget organs from receiving radiation therapy.

computerized tomography: (Also CT scan). Ring-shaped x-ray device used to record computerized "slices" of the body.

core biopsy: Type of biopsy in which needle cuts cylindrically shaped core from target tissue

corpora amylacea: (Also prostatic concretions). Tiny bodies of solidified prostatic fluid that can obstruct the excretory ducts.

corticotrophin-releasing hormone (CRH): Substance produced by the hypothalamus and which is responsible for stimulating the pituitary into secreting ACTH.

Cowper's gland: (See bulbourethral gland).

cryosurgical ablation: Experimental technology using liquid nitrogen to freeze cancer cells.

cystoscopy: Procedure in which specialized telescope is inserted into the bladder through the urethra.

detrusor: Muscle of the bladder.

differentiation: Closeness with which cancer cells resemble normal cells of an organ. A measurement of the aggressiveness and malignant potential of a tumor.

digital rectal examination (DRE): Examination of the rectum and prostate with a gloved finger.

dihydrotestosterone (DHT): Active form of testosterone.

DNA flow cytometry: New technology using an argon laser to examine chromosomes of cancer cells

dorsal vein: Large vein of prostate and penis responsible for most bleeding that occurred in earlier prostate surgery.

dysuria: Painful urination.

ejaculatory duct: One of two channels carrying semen from seminal vesicles to urethra.

enuresis: Bedwetting.

epididymus: One of two small oblong bodies resting on the back of the testes and containing multiple tubular channels carrying sperm from testes to the vas deferens.

estrogen: A female hormone.

eunuch: A male who was castrated prior to onset of puberty.

excretory duct: One of multiple channels carrying prostatic fluid from acini of the prostate to urethra.

external beam radiation: (Also teletherapy). Form of radiation therapy in which energy is delivered from x-ray source outside the body.

external meatus: Opening at end of penis where semen and urine exit through urethra.

external sphincter: Band of muscle downstream from internal sphincter responsible for maintaining urinary continence.

fast neutrons: New, high-energy form of external beam radiation.

fine-needle aspiration (FNA): Form of biopsy in which cell sample is drawn through thin needle rather than taking a piece of target tissue.

flare effect: Initial worsening of symptoms occuring in hormonal therapy with LHRH agonists due to brief increase in production of androgens.

Foley catheter: Thin rubber tube with a balloon at one end inserted into bladder through urethra to drain it of urine.

frequency: Abnormally frequent urination.

frozen section: Rapid diagnostic study of surgically removed specimen used to help the surgeon decide whether an operation should continue.

Gleason system: Most frequently used grading system in prostate cancer.

grade: Measure of degree of differentiation or aggressiveness of a tumor.

gynecomastia: Formation of breasts in a male, a side effect of some prostate cancer treatment methods.

hematuria: Blood in urine.

hesitancy: Increase in length of time between initiation of urination by relaxation of urethral sphincter and when urine stream actually begins.

hyperthermia: Experimental form of treatment where heat is applied to the prostate to kill cancer cells.

hypothalamus: Portion of the brain responsible for controlling many metabolic functions and secretions of numerous endocrine glands.

incidence: Number of new cases of disease arising in a population during a certain period.

incomplete voiding: Desire to urinate immediately after already doing so.

induration: Hardening of an organ. In the prostate gland, often the first objective sign of cancer.

intermittency: Interruption of urinary stream while voiding.

internal sphincter: Band of muscle surrounding urethra as it exits bladder and enters prostate, preventing backward flow of semen during ejaculation.

intravenous pyelography (IVP): Diagnostic study in which dye is injected intravenously and x-ray is taken of urinary tract.

irritative symptoms: Symptoms indirectly related to obstruction of BPH.

laparoscopic pelvic lymph node dissection (PLND): Procedure in which the lymph nodes of the groin are sampled using special telescopic device.

luteinizing hormone (LH): Chemical produced by pituitary gland. Responsible for signalling testes to release testosterone.

luteinizing hormone-releasing hormone (LHRH): Chemical produced by hypothalamus. Responsible for stimulating pituitary into secreting LH.

luteinizing hormone-releasing hormone (LHRH) agonist: Hormonal therapy agent used to effect medical rather than surgical castration.

magnetic resonance imaging (MRI): Tunnel-shaped magnetic device that takes detailed computerized "slices" through the body. (Similar to **CT scan**)

main prostatic gland: Largest of three prostatic gland types. Found mostly in peripheral zone.

malignant: Tending toward metastasis.

membranous urethra: Portion of urethra contained within urogenital diaphragm.

metastasis: Collection of cancer cells that has spread from original tumor site to distant location.

mortality: Number of deaths caused by a disease.

mucosal gland: Smallest of three prostatic gland types. Found mostly in transition and periurethral zones.

neoadjuvant therapy: (Also endocrine downstaging). Technique where hormonal therapy shrinks a tumor before surgery or radiation therapy begins.

neoplasm: New and abnormal growth or tumor.

nerve-sparing radical prostatectomy: Technique where prostate is removed with the intent of preserving erectile function.

neurovascular bundle: Structure responsible for erections, deliberately preserved in nerve-sparing radical prostatectomy.

nocturia: Being awakened in middle of night by urge to void.

nonsteroidal antiandrogen: New type of hormonal therapy agent that prevents binding of male hormone to its target and allows for preservation of sexual function in most cases.

obstructive symptoms: Symptoms of BPH directly related to its squeezing effect on urethra

orchiectomy: (Also castration). Surgical removal or medical removal of testicular function.

palliative: Therapy instituted for symptomatic relief not curative purposes.

Pelvic lymph node dissection (PLND): Surgical procedure in which sample of groin lymph nodes is taken.

penile urethra: Portion of urethra contained within penis.

perineal approach: Surgical technique in which incision is made in perineum.

perineum: Area between scrotum and anus.

peripheral zone: Region of prostate where cancer most commonly appears.

periurethral zone: Smallest of four regions of prostate, containing tissue immediately surrounding prostatic urethra.

permanent section: Diagnostic study in which a tissue sample is stained and mounted on microscope slide.

pituitary gland: Pea-sized gland hanging from base of brain that secretes many different hormones.

post-void residual: Amount of urine remaining in bladder after urination.

pressure-flow studies: Diagnostic techniques that measure pressures within bladder and urethra.

prevalence: Number of cases of a disease existing in a population at a given time.

prevention: Strategy in which a disease is halted before its inception instead of treated after forming.

progestins: Type of female hormone.

prostate-specific antigen (PSA): Protein produced only by prostate gland whose level in blood is invaluable in detecting and treating prostate disease.

PSA density (PSAD): PSA blood level divided by volume of prostate gland.

PSA cancer density (PSACD): PSA level multiplied by volume of tumor itself, then divided by volume of entire prostate gland.

PSA velocity (ΔPSA): Rate of change in PSA value over given time.

prostatic concretion: (See corpora amylacea).

prostatic fluid: Component of semen produced by prostate gland.

prostatic intraepithelial neoplasia (PIN): Precancerous condition of prostate closely resembling cancer, but does not cross basal cell layer.

prostatic urethra: Portion of urethra contained within the prostate.

prostatism: Collection of symptoms caused by benign prostatic hyperplasia (BPH); usually divided into obstructive and irritative symptoms.

radioimmunoguided surgery (RIGS): Experimental technique where radioactive-labeled antibody is injected into body and surgeon uses detection device to locate tumor spread.

rectum: Last segment of colon, or large intestine.

relapse: Return of symptoms after a period of disease remission.

remission: Period during which symptoms abate or disappear.

resectoscope: Long, thin, telescope-like instrument that performs transurethral resection of the prostate (TURP).

retrograde ejaculation: Backward flow of semen during ejaculation.

retropubic approach: Surgical technique where an incision is made between navel and pubic area.

risk factor: Quality that makes a person more susceptible to a specific disease.

salvage surgery: Surgery performed to improve results of a failed primary method.

sarcoma: Cancer arising in skeletal building blocks, like bone, muscle, cartilage, and fibrous tissue.

screening: Testing people in general population who have no symptoms to identify those more likely to have a given disease.

seminal vesicles: Paired structures located behind and above prostate, responsible for producing seminal fluid.

seminiferous tubules: Tiny tubular structures within the testes that produce sperm.

sensitivity: Test ability to select people carrying a given disease from a crowd.

septum (pl. septa): One of several fibrous partitions extending from verumontanum in center of prostate to capsule outside the gland.

silent prostatism: BPH obstruction without symptoms.

simulation: Phase of radiation therapy when oncologist customizes according to the individual body and tumor the area that will receive radiation.

specificity: Ability of test to detect disease of interest and ignore other diseases.

stage: Degree of spread of tumor.

staging: Process in which tests and procedures are performed to determine stage of a given tumor.

stent: Flexible, tube-shaped metal coil or mesh inserted into prostatic urethra to hold it open.

steroid synthesis blocker: Any of a number of drugs for other medical conditions, but which can block production of androgens by adrenal glands.

strangury: Pain at end of urination.

stress incontinence: Involuntary leakage of urine occuring at times of increased bladder pressure, such as lifting or coughing.

submucosal gland: Intermediate-sized prostatic gland type, surrounding mucosal gland region.

template: Metal plate with holes assisting placement of interstitial radioactive implants.

terminal dribbling: Low-level flow for several seconds at end of urination

testosterone: Male hormone produced by Leydig cells of the testes; necessary for growth and development of normal and cancerous prostate cells.

Texas catheter: (Also condom catheter). Urinary drainage system where a tube with condom-like endpiece covers penis.

thermal therapy: Experimental treatment for BPH where microwave probe heats prostate to temperatures over 45°C (113°F).

TNM system: Staging system frequently used in malignancies of other organs, but infrequently in prostate cancer.

transition zone: Region of prostate where benign prostatic hyperplasia (BPH) most commonly appears.

transrectal ultrasound (TRUS): Diagnostic procedure where probe is inserted in rectum and computerized pictures are taken of prostate using sound waves.

transurethral incision of the prostate (TUIP): Surgical procedure where prostatic tissue is cut, not removed.

transurethral resection of the prostate (TURP): Surgical procedure where prostatic tissue is removed with an instrument called resectoscope inserted through urethra.

TURP syndrome: Collection of symptoms, including mental confusion, nausea and vomiting, high blood pressure, slow heart rate, and vision changes, following a small number of TURPs and occurring when irrigation fluid used during the procedure is inadvertently absorbed into bloodstream.

ureter: Tube carrying urine from kidney to bladder.

urethra: Tube carrying urine and semen outside the body. Divided into prostatic, membranous, and penile segments.

urgency: Overwhelming need to urinate, often accompanied by sensation that leakage or urge incontinence will occur if need isn't satisfied.

uroflowmetry: Diagnostic test measuring flow rate of the urinary stream.

urogenital diaphragm: Sheet of muscle composing pelvic floor.

utricle: Embryologic remnant that is smallest of male accessory glands.

vas deferens: One of two ducts carrying sperm and semen from epididymus to ejaculatory ducts.

vasectomy: Male sterilization procedure where vas deferens is divided, preventing sperm from traveling from testes to penis.

verumontanum: Elevation on back wall of urethra where prostatic utricle, ejaculatory ducts, and excretory ducts end. Also called colliculus seminalis.

Whitmore-Jewett system: Most frequently used staging system in prostate cancer.

BIBLIOGRAPHY

Chapter 1

AMENTA, P. 1987. *Elias-Pauly's Histology and Human Micro-anatomy.* New York. John Wiley & Sons.

BLANDY, J., AND B. LYTTON. 1986. *The Prostate.* Kent, England. Butterworths.

CORMACK, D. 1984. *Introduction to Histology.* Philadelphia. J. B. Lippincott.

FAWCETT, D. 1986. *A Textbook of Histology.* Philadelphia. W. B. Saunders.

FITZPATRICK, J., AND R. KRANE. 1989. *The Prostate.* New York. Churchill Livingstone.

GENESER, F. 1986. *Textbook of Histology.* Philadelphia. Lea & Febiger.

GUYTON, A. 1981. *Textbook of Medical Physiology.* Philadelphia. W. B. Saunders.

KELLY, D., ET AL. 1984. *Bailey's Textbook of Microscopic Anatomy.* Baltimore. Williams & Wilkins.

VICK, R. 1984. *Contemporary Medical Physiology.* Menlo Park, CA. Addison-Wesley.

Chapter 2

BERKOW, R., ET AL., ED. 1987. *The Merck Manual.* Rahway, NJ. Merck Sharp & Dohme Research Laboratories.

BRAUNWALD, E., ET AL., ED. 1987. *Harrison's Principles of Internal Medicine.* New York. McGraw-Hill.

BRUCE, A., AND J. TRACHTENBERG, EDS. 1987. *Adenocarcinoma of the Prostate.* New York. Springer-Verlag.

CATALONA, W. 1984. *Prostate Cancer.* Orlando, FL. Grune & Stratton.

DAS, S., AND E. D. CRAWFORD, EDS. 1993. *Cancer of the Prostate.* New York. Marcel Dekker.

PRESIDENT'S CANCER PANEL MEETING. 1992. Bethesda, MD. National Institutes of Health: National Cancer Institute.

RAMSEY, P., AND E. LARSON. 1993. *Medical Therapeutics.* Philadelphia. W. B. Saunders.

SCHWARTZ, S., ET AL., ED. 1989. *Principles of Surgery.* New York. McGraw-Hill.

SMITH, J. AND R. MIDDLETON. 1987. *Clinical Management of Prostatic Carcinoma.* Chicago. Year Book Medical Publishing.

WALSH, P., ET AL., ED. 1992. *Campbell's Urology.* Philadelphia. W.B. Saunders.

Chapter 3

BABAIAN, R. J., AND J. CAMPS. 1991. "The Role of PSA as Part of a Diagnostic Triad and as a Guide When to Perform a Biopsy." *Cancer.* 68(9): 2060-2063.

BERKOW, R., ET AL., ED. 1987. *The Merck Manual.* Rahway, NJ. Merck Sharp & Dohme Research Laboratories.

BRAUNWALD, E., ET AL., ED. 1987. *Harrison's Principles of Internal Medicine.* New York. McGraw-Hill.

CATALONA, W. 1984. *Prostate Cancer.* Orlando, FL. Grune & Stratton.

DAS, S., AND E. D. CRAWFORD, EDS. 1993. *Cancer of the Prostate.* New York. Marcel Dekker.

DJAVAN, B., AND C. ROEHRBORN. 1994. "Prostate-Specific Antigen: When to Measure It—How to Interpret Results." *Consultant.* 34(6): 909–916.

DOUBLET, J. 1994. "Laparoscopic Pelvic Lymph Node Dissection for Staging of Prostatic Cancer." *European Urology.* 25(3): 194–198.

DYKE, C. 1990. "Value of Random Ultrasound-Guided Transrectal Prostate Biopsy." *Radiology.* 176(2): 345–349.

FORSSLUND, G., ET AL. 1992. "The Prognostic Significance of Nuclear DNA Content in Prostatic Carcinoma." *Cancer.* 69(6): 1432–1439.

GLENN, J., ED. 1991. *Urologic Surgery.* Philadelphia. J. B. Lippincott.

GRUPS, J. W., ET AL. 1990. "Diagnostic Value of Transrectal Ultrasound in Tumor Staging and in Detection of Incidental Prostatic Cancer." *Urologie Internationalis.* 45(1): 38–40.

HANKS, G. 1993. "The Challenge of Treating Node-Positive Prostate Cancer." *Cancer.* 71(3 suppl.): 1014–1018.

HONIG, S. 1992. "The Role of Fine-Needle Aspiration Biopsy of the Prostate in Staging Adenocarcinoma." *Cancer.* 69(12): 2978–2982.

HUSSAIN, M., ET AL. 1993. "Flow Cytometric DNA Analysis of Fresh Prostatic Resections." *Cancer.* 72(10): 3012–3019.

KAVOUISSI, L. 1994. "Editorial: Techniques for Nodal Staging in Prostate Cancer." *Journal of Urology.* 151(5): 1324–1325.

MAZEMAN, E., et al. 1992. "Extraperitoneal Pelvioscopy in Lymph Node Staging of Bladder and Prostatic Cancer." *Journal of Urology.* 147(2): 366–370.

MCDOWELL, G., et al. 1990. "Pelvic Lymphadenectomy for Staging Clinically Localized Prostate Cancer." *Urology.* 35(6): 476–482.

METTLIN, C. 1993. "American Cancer Society—National Prostate Cancer Detection Project." *Cancer.* 71(3): 891–898.

PALKEN, M., et al. 1990. "Prostate Cancer: Correlation of DRE, TRUS, and PSA levels with Tumor Volume in Radical Prostatectomy Specimens." *Journal of Urology.* 143(6): 1155–1162.

RIFKIN, M., ET AL. 1991. "Palpable Masses in the Prostate: Superior Accuracy of Ultrasound-Guided Biopsy Compared with Accuracy of Digitally Guided Biopsy." *Radiology.* 179(1): 41–42.

SCHIEBLER, M. L., ET AL. 1991. "Comparison of Digital Rectal Examination, Endorectal Ultrasound, Body Coil MRI in Staging of Adenocarcinoma of the Prostate." *Urologic Radiology.* 13(2): 110–118.

SCHMIDT, J. 1992. "Clinical Diagnosis of Prostate Cancer." *Cancer*. 70(1): 221–224.

SCHUESSLER, W., ET AL. 1991. "Transperitoneal Endosurgical Lymphadenectomy in Patients With Localized Prostate Cancer." *Journal of Urology*. 145(5): 988–991.

SCHWARTZ, S., ET AL., ED. 1989. *Principles of Surgery*. New York. McGraw-Hill.

SMITH, J., AND R. MIDDLETON. 1987. *Clinical Management of Prostatic Carcinoma*. Chicago. Year Book Medical Publishing.

TINARI, N., ET AL. 1993. "DNA and S-Phase Fraction Analysis by Flow Cytometry in Prostate Cancer." *Cancer*. 71(4): 1289–1296.

WALSH, P., ET AL., ED. 1992. *Campbell's Urology*. Philadelphia. W.B. Saunders.

Chapter 4

ANDRIOLE, G., AND W. CATALONA. 1993. "Using PSA to Screen for Prostate Cancer." *Urologic Clinics of North America*. 20(4): 647–651.

ARAI, Y. 1990. "Value of PSA Measurements in Predicting Lymph Node Involvement in Prostatic Carcinoma." *Urologia Internationalis*. 45(6): 356–360.

BJARTELL, A., ET AL. 1993. "Production of Alpha-1-Antichymotrypsin by PSA-Containing Cells of Human Prostate Epithelium." *Urology*. 42(5): 502–508.

BJŠRK, T., ET AL. 1994. "Alpha-1-Antichymotrypsin Production in PSA-Producing Cells Is Common in Prostatic Carcinoma but Rare in BPH." *Urology*. 43(4): 427–433.

BLACKWELL, K., ET AL. 1994. "Combining PSA with Cancer and Gland Volume to Predict More Reliably Pathological Stage: The Influence of PSA Cancer Density." *Journal of Urology*. 151(6): 1565–1570.

CADEDDU, J., ET AL. 1993. "Relationship Between Changes in Prostate Specific Antigen and Prognosis of Prostate Cancer." *Urology*. 42(4): 383–389.

CARTER, H. B. 1994. "Current Status of Prostate-Specific Antigen in the Management of Prostate Cancer." *Advances in Surgery*. 27: 81–95.

CARTER, H. B., AND J. PEARSON. 1993. "PSA Velocity for the Diagnosis of Early Prostate Cancer." *Urologic Clinics of North America.* 20(4): 665–670.

COCKETT, A. 1993. "Treatment Strategies for Prostate Cancer." *Journal of the American Medical Association.* 270(14): 1692.

CRAWFORD, E. D., AND E. DEANTONI. 1993. "Prostate-Specific Antigen as a Screening Test for Prostate Cancer." *Urologic Clinics of North America.* 20(4): 637–645.

DISILVERIO, F., ET AL. 1992. "New Ultrasensitive Assay Developed by Using Monoclonal Antibodies for Detecting Prostate-Specific Antigen." *European Urology.* 21(suppl 1): 79–82.

DJAVAN, B., AND C. ROEHRBORN. 1994. "Prostate-Specific Antigen: When to Measure It—How to Interpret Results." *Consultant.* 34(6): 909–916.

DORR, V., ET AL. 1993. "An Evaluation of Prostate-Specific Antigen as a Screening Test for Prostate Cancer." *Archives of Internal Medicine.* 153(22): 2529–2537.

GOAD, J., ET AL. 1993. "PSA After Definitive Radiotherapy for Clinically Localized Prostate Cancer." *Urologic Clinics of North America.* 20(4): 727–735.

GUESS, H., ET AL. 1993. "The Effect of Finasteride on Prostate-Specific Antigen in Men with Benign Prostatic Hyperplasia. *The Prostate.* 22(1): 31–37.

———. 1993. "Effect of Finasteride on Serum Prostate-Specific Antigen Concentration in Men With Benign Prostatic Hyperplasia." *Urologic Clinics of North America.* 20(4): 627–635.

KLEER, E., AND J. OESTERLING. 1993. "Prostate-Specific Antigen and Staging of Localized Prostate Carcinoma." *Urologic Clinics of North America.* 20(4): 695–704.

LANGE, P. 1993. "Screening with Prostate-Specific Antigen: Should We or Shouldn't We?" *Journal of the American Medical Association.* 269(17): 2212.

LEINONEN, J., ET AL. 1993. "Double-Label Time-Resolved Immunofluorometric Assay of PSA and of its Complex with Alpha-1-Antichymotrypsin." *Clinical Chemistry.* 39(10): 2098–2102.

LILJA, H. 1993. "Significance of Different Molecular Forms of Serum Prostate-Specific Antigen." *Urologic Clinics of North America*. 20(4): 681–685.

OESTERLING, J., ET AL. 1993. "Influence of Patient Age on the Serum Prostate-Specific Antigen." *Urologic Clinics of North America*. 20(4): 671–679.

OESTERLING, J. 1993. "Using Prostate-Specific Antigen to Eliminate the Staging Radionuclide Bone Scan." *Urologic Clinics of North America*. 20(4): 705–711.

PARTIN, A., ET AL. 1993. "Serum PSA After Anatomic Radical Prostatectomy." *Urologic Clinics of North America*. 20(4): 713–724.

PETROS, J., AND G. ANDRIOLE. 1993. "Serum PSA After Antiandrogen Therapy." *Urologic Clinics of North America*. 20(4): 749–755.

PRESIDENT'S CANCER PANEL MEETING. 1992. Bethesda, MD. National Institutes of Health: National Cancer Institute.

SEAMAN, E., ET AL. 1993. "PSA Density (PSAD)." *Urologic Clinics of North America*. 20(4): 653–663.

SEMJONOW, A., ET AL. 1994. "Prostate-Specific Antigen Corrected for Prostate Volume Improves Differentiation of Benign Prostatic Hyperplasia and Organ-Confined Prostatic Carcinoma." *British Journal of Urology*. 73(5): 538–543.

SHEARER, R. J. 1993. "Prostate-Specific Antigen." *The Lancet*. 342(8876): 903.

STAMEY, T., ET AL. 1993. "Early Detection of Residual Prostate Cancer After Radical Prostatectomy by an Ultrasensitive Assay for PSA." *Journal of Urology*. 149(4): 787–792.

WALSH, P., ET AL., ED. 1992. *Campbell's Urology*. Philadelphia. W. B. Saunders.

WALSH, P. 1993. "Using Prostate-Specific Antigen to Diagnose Prostate Cancer: Sailing in Uncharted Waters." *Annals of Internal Medicine*. 119(9): 948–949.

ZAGARS, G. "Serum PSA as a Tumor Marker for Patients Undergoing Definitive Radiation Therapy." *Urologic Clinics of North America*. 20(4): 737–746.

ZENTNER, P., ET AL. 1993. "PSAD: A New Prognostic Indicator for Prostate Cancer." *International Journal of Radiation Oncology, Biology, and Physics*. 27(1): 47–58.

Chapter 5

ANDRIOLE, G., AND W. CATALONA. 1994. "Prostate Carcinoma." *Annual Review of Medicine*. 45: 351–359.

BADALAMENT, R., ET AL. 1993. "Radioimmunoguided Radical Prostatectomy and Lymphadenectomy." *Cancer*. 71(7): 2268–2275.

CATALONA, W. 1992. "Radical Surgery for Advanced Prostate Cancer and for Radiation Failures." *Journal of Urology*. 147(3 pt. 2): 916.

———. 1994. "PSA and the Detection of Prostate Cancer." *Journal of the American Medical Association*. 271(3): 192.

CHENG, C. 1993. "Stage D1 Prostate Cancer." *Cancer*. 71(3 suppl.): 996–1004.

EKMAN, P. 1993. "Dilemma of Microscopic Lymph Node Metastases in Human Prostate Cancer. *European Urology*. 24(suppl. 2): 57–60.

"FDA Approves Implant to Treat Incontinence." 10/5/93. *The Washington Post*.

FOWLER, J., ED. 1992 *Urologic Surgery*. Boston. Little, Brown.

GLENN, J., ED. 1991. *Urologic Surgery*. Philadelphia. J. B. Lippincott.

HANKS, G. E. 1991. "Radiotherapy or Surgery for Prostate Cancer?" *Acta Oncologica*. 30(2): 231–237.

———. 1993. "The Challenge of Treating Node Positive Prostate Cancer." *Cancer*. 71(3 suppl.): 1014–1018.

LERNER, S., ET AL. 1994. "Combined Laparoscopic Pelvic Lymph Node Dissection and Modified Belt Radical Perineal Prostatectomy for Localized Prostatic Adenocarcinoma." *Urology*. 43(4): 493–497.

LU-YAO, G., AND E. R. GREENBERG. 1994. "Changes in Prostate Cancer Incidence and Treatment in the USA." *Lancet*. 343(8892): 251–254.

MACALUSO, J., ET AL. 1994. "Transperineal Percutaneous Radical Cryosurgical Ablation of the Prostate Under Transrectal Ultrasound Guidance for Treatment of Carcinoma of the Prostate." *Journal of the Louisiana State Medical Society*. 146(1): 18–24.

MONTIE, J. 1993. "Counseling the Patient with Regional Metastasis of Prostate Cancer." *Cancer.* 71(3 suppl.): 1019–1023.

MORGAN, W., et al. 1993 "Long-Term Evaluation of Radical Prostatectomy as Treatment for Clinical Stage C Prostate Cancer." *Urology.* 41(2): 113–120.

MOUL, J., AND D. PAULSON. 1991. "The Role of Radical Surgery in the Management of Radiation Recurrent and Large Volume Prostate Cancer." *Cancer.* 68(6): 1265–1271.

NARAYAN, P. 1994. "Neoadjuvant Hormonal Therapy and Radical Prostatectomy for Clinical Stage C Carcinoma of the Prostate." *British Journal of Urology.* 73(5): 544–548.

PARKINS, T. 1994. "Concern Grows Over Prostate Cancer Treatment Options." *Journal of the National Cancer Institute.* 86(12): 897–898.

PETROVICH, Z. "Radiotherapy Following Radical Prostatectomy in Patients with Adenocarcinoma of the Prostate." *International Journal of Radiation Oncology, Biology, and Physics.* 21(4): 949–954.

PONTES, J. E. 1993. "Salvage Surgery for Radiation Failure in Prostate Cancer." *Cancer.* 71(3 suppl.): 976–980.

PRESIDENT'S CANCER PANEL MEETING. 1992. Bethesda, MD. National Institutes of Health: National Cancer Institute.

RAMON, J., ET AL. 1993. "Urinary Continence Following Radical Retropubic Prostatectomy. *British Journal of Urology.* 71(1): 47–51.

SCHOVER, L. 1993. "Sexual Rehabilitation After Treatment for Prostate Cancer." *Cancer.* 71(3 suppl.): 1024–1030.

SCHULMAN, C. C., AND A. M. SASSINE. 1993. "Neoadjuvant Hormonal Deprivation Before Radical Prostatectomy." *European Urology.* 24(4): 450–455.

SOLE-BALCELLS, F. 1992. "Post-surgical Management of the Patient Undergoing Radical Prostatectomy. *British Journal of Urology.* 70(suppl. 1): 43–49.

SOLOWAY, M. S. 1993. "Significance of Androgen Deprivation Prior to Radical Prostatectomy with Special Reference to PSA." *World Journal of Urology.* 11(4): 221–226.

STEIN, A. 1992. "Adjuvant Radiotherapy in Patients Post-Radical Prostatectomy with Tumor Extending Through Capsule or Positive Seminal Vesicles." *Urology.* 39(1): 59–62.

———. 1992. "Salvage Radical Prostatectomy After Failure of Curative Radiotherapy for Adenocarcinoma of the Prostate." *Urology.* 40(3): 197–200.

TELANG, D., et al. 1992. "Radical Surgery in the Treatment of Localized Cancer of the Prostate." *Henry Ford Hospital Medical Journal.* 40(1&2): 108–110.

WALSH, P., ET AL. 1990. "Preservation of Sexual Function in Men During Radical Pelvic Surgery." *Maryland Medical Journal.* 39(4): 389–393.

WASSON, J., ET AL. 1993. "A Structured Literature Review of Treatment for Localized Prostate Cancer." *Archives of Family Medicine.* 2(5): 487–493.

ZIETMAN, A. L., ET AL. 1993. "Adjuvant Irradiation After Radical Prostatectomy for Adenocarcinoma of the Prostate: Analysis of Freedom from PSA Failure." *Urology.* 42(3): 292–297.

———. 1993. "Residual Disease After Radical Surgery or Radiation Therapy for Prostate Cancer." *Cancer.* 71(3 suppl.): 959–969.

ZINCKE, H. 1992. "Stage D1 Prostate Cancer Treated with Radical Prostatectomy and Adjuvant Hormonal Therapy." Cancer. 70 (1 suppl.): 311–323.

Chapter 6

BAGSHAW, M., ET AL. 1993. "Radiation Therapy for Localized Disease." *Cancer.* 71(3 suppl.): 939–952.

ENNIS, R., AND R. PESCHEL. 1993. "Radiation Therapy for Prostate Cancer." *Cancer.* 72(9): 2644-2650.

EPSTEIN, B., AND G. HANKS. 1992. "Prostate Cancer: Evaluation and Radiotherapeutic Management." *CA: A Cancer Journal for Clinicians.* 42(4): 223–239.

JENRETTE, J., AND L. HARRELL. 1994. "Prostate Cancer: The Role of Radiation Therapy." *Journal of the South Carolina Medical Association.* 90(5): 222–224.

KHIL, M., AND J. KIM. 1992. "Therapeutic Options for Localized Carcinoma of the Prostate: The Role of External Beam Radiation Therapy." *Henry Ford Hospital Medical Journal.* 40(1-2): 103–106.

KLEINBERG, L. 1994. "Treatment-Related Symptoms During the First Year Following Transperineal 125I Prostate Implantation." *International Journal of Radiation Oncology, Biology, and Physics.* 28(4): 985–990.

KOPROWSKI, C. 1992. "Response to Drs. Peschel and Wallner." *International Journal of Radiation Oncology, Biology, and Physics.* 23(1): 254.

LANNON, S. G., ET AL. 1993. "Long-Term Results of Combined Interstitial Gold Seed Implantation and External Beam Irradiation in Localized Cancer of the Prostate." *British Journal of Urology.* 72(5): 782–791.

LARAMORE, G. E. 1993. "Fast Neutron Radiotherapy for Locally Advanced Prostate Cancer." *American Journal of Clinical Oncology.* 16(2): 164–167.

LOENING, S., AND J. W. TURNER. 1993. "Use of Percutaneous Transperineal 198Au Seeds to Treat Recurrent Prostate Adenocarcinoma After Failure of Definitive Radiotherapy." *The Prostate.* 23(4): 283–290.

MILLER, E. B., ET AL. 1993. "Re-evaluation of Prostate Biopsy After Definitive Radiation Therapy." *Urology.* 41(4): 311–316.

MONTORSI, F., ET AL. 1992. "Transrectal Microwave Hyperthermia for Advanced Prostate Cancer: Long-Term Clinical Results." *Journal of Urology.* (2 pt. 1): 342–345.

PEREZ, C. 1993. "Irradiation in Relapsing Carcinoma of the Prostate." *Cancer.* 71(3 suppl.): 1110–1122.

PEREZ, P., ET AL. 1993. "Localized Carcinoma of the Prostate." *Cancer.* 72(11): 3156–3173.

PESCHEL, R. 1992. "Iodine$_{125}$ Implants for Prostate Cancer." *International Journal of Radiation Oncology, Biology, and Physics.* 23(1): 254.

PRESIDENT'S CANCER PANEL MEETING. 1992. Bethesda, MD. National Institutes of Health: National Cancer Institute.

PRESTIDGE, B., ET AL. 1992. "The Clinical Significance of Positive Post-Irradiation Prostatic Biopsy Without Metastases." *International Journal of Radiation Oncology, Biology, and Physics.* 24(3): 403–408.

———. 1994. "Predictors of Survival After Positive Post-Irradiation Prostate Biopsy." *International Journal of Radiation Oncology, Biology, and Physics.* 28(1): 17–22.

PRIONAS, S., ET AL. 1994. "Thermometry of Interstitial Hyperthermia Given as an Adjuvant to Brachytherapy for Treatment of Carcinoma of the Prostate." *International Journal of Radiation Oncology, Biology, and Physics.* 28(1): 151–162.

ROACH, M., ET AL. 1994. "Defining Treatment Margins for Six-Field Conformal Irradiation of Localized Prostate Cancer." *International Journal of Radiation Oncology, Biology, and Physics.* 28(1): 267–275.

RUSSELL, K., ET AL. 1994. "Photon vs. Fast Neutron External Beam Radiotherapy in the Treatment of Locally Advanced Prostate Cancer: Results of a Randomized Prospective Trial." *International Journal of Radiation Oncology, Biology, and Physics.* 28(1): 47–54.

SERVADIO, C., AND Z. LEIB. 1991. "Local Hyperthermia for Prostate Cancer." *Urology.* 38(4): 307–309.

STAWARZ, B. 1993 "Transrectal Hyperthermia as Palliative Treatment for Advanced Adenocarcinoma of the Prostate and Studies of Cell-Mediated Immunity." *Urology.* 41(6): 548–553.

STROMBERG, J., ET AL. 1994 "Improved Local Control and Survival for Surgically Staged Patients with Locally Advanced Prostate Cancer Treated with Up-Front Low-Dose 192I Prostate Implantation and External Beam Irradiation." *International Journal of Radiation Oncology, Biology, and Physics.* 28(1): 67–75.

WEYRICH, T., ET AL. 1993. "125I Seed Implants for Prostatic Carcinoma." *Urology.* 41(2): 122–125.

ZAGARS, G. 1993. "Prognostic Factors in Prostate Cancer." *Cancer.* 72(5): 1709–1725.

Chapter 7

AFRIN, L., AND R. STUART. 1994. "Medical Therapy of Prostate Cancer." *Journal of the South Carolina Medical Association.* 90(5): 231–236.

BENSON, R. 1992. "A Rationale for the Use of Non-steroidal Anti-androgens in the Management of Prostate Cancer." *The Prostate.* Suppl. 4: 85–90.

COOKSON, M., AND M. SAROSDY. 1994. "Hormonal Therapy for Metastatic Prostate Cancer." *Southern Medical Journal.* 87(1): 1–6.

DANESHGARI, F., AND E. D. CRAWFORD. 1993. "Endocrine Therapy of Advanced Carcinoma of the Prostate." *Cancer.* 71(3 suppl.): 1089–1097.

DENIS, L. 1993. "Prostate Cancer." *Cancer.* 71(3 suppl.): 1050–1058.

FRANCINI, G., ET AL. 1993. "Weekly Chemotherapy in Advanced Prostate Cancer." *British Journal of Cancer.* 67(6): 1430–1436.

GORMLEY, G. 1991. "Role of 5-alpha-Reductase Inhibitors in the Treatment of Advanced Prostatic Carcinoma." *Urologic Clinics of North America.* 18(1): 93–97.

GUDZIAK, M., AND A. SMITH. 1994. "Hormonal Therapy for Stage D Cancer of the Prostate." *Western Journal of Medicine.* 160(4): 351–359.

HERR, H., ET AL. 1993. "A Comparison of the Quality of Life of Patients with Metastatic Prostate Cancer Who Received or Did Not Receive Hormonal Therapy." *Cancer.* 71(3 suppl.): 1143–1150.

KOZLOWSKI, J., ET AL. 1991. "Advanced Prostatic Carcinoma." *Urologic Clinics of North America.* 18(1): 15–22.

LABRIE, F., ET AL. 1993. "Combination Therapy for Prostate Cancer." *Cancer.* 71(3 suppl.): 1059–1067.

LEO, M., ET AL. 1991. "PSA in Hormonally Treated Stage D2 Prostate Cancer: Is It Always an Accurate Indicator of Disease Status?" *Journal of Urology.* 145(4): 802–806.

MATZKIN, H., AND M. SOLOWAY. 1992. "Response to Second-Line Hormonal Manipulation Monitored by Serum PSA in Stage D2 Prostate Carcinoma." *Urology.* 40(1): 78–80.

MATZKIN, H., ET AL. 1993. "Relapse on Endocrine Treatment in Patients with Stage D2 Prostate Cancer." *Urology.* 41(2): 144–148.

McLEOD, D. 1993. "Antiandrogenic Drugs." *Cancer.* 71(3 suppl.): 1046–1049.

MILLER, J., ET AL. 1992. "The Clinical Usefulness of Serum PSA After Hormonal Therapy of Metastatic Prostate Cancer." *Journal of Urology.* 147(3 pt. 2): 956–961.

SCHER H., AND W. K. KELLY. 1993. "Flutamide Withdrawal Syndrome: Its Impact on Clinical Trials in Hormone-Refractory Prostate Cancer." *Journal of Clinical Oncology.* 11(8): 1566–1572.

SCHLEGEL, P. N. 1994. "Medical Management of Prostatic Diseases." *Advances in Internal Medicine.* 39: 586–597.

SMALL, E. 1994. "Hormonal Therapy for Metastatic Prostate Cancer." *Western Journal of Medicine.* 160(3): 253–254.

YAGODA, A., AND D. PETRYLAK. 1993. "Cytotoxic Chemotherapy for Advanced Hormone-Resistant Prostate Cancer." *Cancer.* 71(3 suppl.): 1098–1109.

ZELEFSKY, M., ET AL. 1994. "Neoadjuvant Hormonal Therapy Improves the Therapeutic Ratio in Patients with Bulky Prostatic Cancer Treated with 3D Conformal Radiation Therapy." *International Journal of Radiation Oncology, Biology, and Physics.* 29(4): 755–761.

Chapter 8

ADOLFSSON, J. 1991. "Deferred Therapy in Well and Moderately Differentiated Prostate Cancer." *Acta Oncologica.* 30(2): 225–226.

BRAWER, M. 1992. "Prostatic Intraepithelial Neoplasia: A Premalignant Lesion." *Journal of Clinical Biochemistry.* Suppl. 16G: 171–174.

CATALONA, W. 1993. "Treatment Strategies for Prostate Cancer." *Journal of the American Medical Association.* 270(14): 1692.

CHODAK, G. W., ET AL. 1994. "Results of Conservative Management of Clinically Localized Prostate Cancer." *New England Journal of Medicine.* 330(4): 242–248.

COCKETT, A. 1993. "Treatment Strategies for Prostate Cancer." *Journal of the American Medical Association.* 270(14): 1692.

COFFEY, D., ET AL. 1987. *Current Concepts and Approaches to the Study of Prostate Cancer.* New York. Alan R. Liss, Inc.

DE LA TORRE, M., ET AL. 1993. "Prostatic Intraepithelial Neoplasia and Invasive Carcinoma in Total Prostatectomy Specimens: Distribution, Volumes, and DNA Ploidy." *British Journal of Urology.* 72: 207–213.

ELLIS, W., AND M. BRAWER. 1993. "Prostate-Specific Antigen in Benign Prostatic Hyperplasia and Prostatic Intraepithelial Neoplasia." *Urologic Clinics of North America.* 20(4): 621–625.

EPSTEIN, J., ET AL. 1994. "Pathologic and Clinical Findings to Predict Tumor Extent of Nonpalpable (Stage T1c) Prostate Cancer." *Journal of the American Medical Association.* 271(5): 368–374.

EPSTEIN, J., ET AL. 1994. "Small High-Grade Adenocarcinoma of the Prostate in Radical Prostatectomy Specimens Performed for Nonpalpable Disease: Pathogenetic and Clinical Implications." *Journal of Urology.* 151(6): 1587–1592.

FAIR, W. 1992. "The Natural History of Locally Confined Prostate Cancer: A Review." *The Prostate.* Suppl. 4: 79–84.

GREEN, L. 1993. "Digital Rectal Examination Screening for Prostate Cancer." *Journal of the American Medical Association.* 270(11): 1315.

MCNEAL, J. 1993. "Prostatic Microcarcinomas in Relation to Cancer Origin and the Evolution to Clinical Cancer." *Cancer.* 71(3 suppl.): 984–991.

PAGANO, F., ET AL. 1991. "Is There a Relationship Between Benign Prostatic Hyperplasia and Prostatic Cancer?" *European Urology.* 20(Suppl. 2): 31–35.

SHARP, J. 1993. "Expanding the Definition of Quality of Life for Prostate Cancer." *Cancer.* 71(3 suppl.): 1078–1082.

STORMONT, T., ET AL. 1993. "Clinical Stage B0 or T1c Prostate Cancer: Nonpalpable D2 Identified by Elevated Serum PSA Concentration." *Urology.* 41(1): 3–8.

WAYMONT, B., ET AL. 1993. "Treatment Preferences of Urologists in Great Britain and Ireland in the Management of Prostate Cancer." *British Journal of Urology.* 71(5): 577–582.

WHITMORE, W. F., ET AL. 1992. "Conservative Management of Localized Prostatic Cancer." *American Journal of Clinical Oncology.* 15(5): 446–452.

WHITTEMORE, A., ET AL. 1991. "Low-Grade, Latent Prostate Cancer Volume: Predictor of Clinical Cancer Incidence." *Journal of the National Cancer Institute.* 83(17): 1231–1235.

ZHANG, G., ET AL. 1991. "Long-Term Followup Results After Expectant Management of Stage A1 Prostatic Cancer." *Journal of Urology.* 146(1): 96–103.

Chapter 9

BOSLAND, M. 1992. "Possible Enhancement of Prostate Carcinogenesis by Some Chemopreventive Agents." *Journal of Cellular Biochemistry.* Suppl. 16H: 135–137.

BRAVO, M. P. 1991. "Dietary Factors and Prostate Cancer." *Urologia Internationales.* 46: 163–166.

BRAWLEY, O., AND I. THOMPSON. 1994. "Chemoprevention of Prostate Cancer." *Urology.* 43(5): 594–597.

CHAMBERLAIN, J., AND J. MELIA. 1993. "Prospects for Prevention." *The Lancet.* 342(8876): 902.

CRAWFORD, ET AL. 1992. "Chemoprevention of Prostate Cancer: Guidelines for Possible Intervention Strategies." *Journal of Cellular Biochemistry.* Suppl. 16H: 140–145.

GELLER, J., AND L. SIONIT. 1992. "Castration-like Effects on the Human Prostate of a 5-α-reductase Inhibitor, Finasteride." *Journal of Cellular Biochemistry.* Suppl. 16H: 109–112.

GORMLEY, G. "Chemoprevention Strategies for Prostate Cancer: The Role of 5-α-reductase Inhibitors." *Journal of Cellular Biochemistry.* Suppl. 16H: 113–117.

HANCHETTE, C., AND G. SCHWARTZ. 1992. "Geographic Patterns of Prostate Cancer Mortality." *Cancer.* 70(12): 2861–2869.

KADMON, D. 1992. "Chemoprevention in Prostate Cancer: The Role of DFMO." *Journal of Cellular Biochemistry.* Suppl. 16H: 122–127.

KELLOFF, G., ET AL. 1992. "Introductory Remarks: Development of Chemopreventive Agents for Prostate Cancer." *Journal of Cellular Biochemistry.* Suppl. 16H: 1–8.

LEE, I. M. 1992. "Physical Activity and Risk of Prostate Cancer Among College Alumni." *American Journal of Epidemiology.* 135(2): 169–179.

LEYTON, J., ET AL. 1994. "Recombinant Human Uteroglobin Inhibits the In Vitro Invasiveness of Human Metastatic Prostate Tumor Cells and the Release of Arachidonic Acid Stimulated by Fibroblast-Conditioned Medium." *Cancer Research.* 54: 3696–3699.

REYNOLDS, T. 1993. "Prostate Cancer Prevention Trial Launched." *Journal of the National Cancer Institute.* 85(20): 1633–1634.

SCHWARTZ, G., AND B. HULKA. 1990. "Is Vitamin D Deficiency a Risk Factor for Prostate Cancer?" *Anticancer Research.* 10: 1307–1312.

WILLIAMS, R., ET AL. 1992. "When is Intervention Warranted?" *Journal of Cellular Biochemistry.* Suppl. 16H: 138–139.

Chapter 10

CALAIS DE SILVA, F. 1993. "Quality of Life in Prostatic Cancer Patients." *Cancer.* 72(12 suppl.): 3803–3806.

PEDERSEN, K. V. 1993. "Quality of Life After Radical Retropubic Prostatectomy for Carcinoma of the Prostate." *European Urology.* 24(1): 7–11.

SHARP, J., ET AL. 1993. "Elderly Men With Cancer: Social Work Interventions in Prostate Cancer." *Social Work in Health Care.* 19(1): 91–105.

SHARP, J. "Expanding the Definition of Quality of Life for Prostate Cancer." *Cancer.* 71(3 suppl.): 1078–1082.

SINGER, P. 1991. "Sex or Survival: Trade-Offs Between Quality and Quantity of Life." *Journal of Clinical Oncology.* 9(2): 328-334.

Chapter 11

FITZPATRICK, J., AND R. KRANE, EDS. 1989. *The Prostate.* London. Churchill Livingstone.

KURTH, K., AND D. NEWLING, EDS. 1994. *EORTC Genitourinary Group Monograph 12: Benign Prostatic Hyperplasia: Recent Progress in Clinical Research and Practice.* New York. Wiley-Liss.

LEPOR, H., AND R. LAWSON, EDS. 1993. *Prostate Diseases.* Philadelphia. W. B. Saunders.

MCCONNELL, J. D., ET AL. 1994. *Benign Prostatic Hyperplasia: Diagnosis and Treatment. Clinical Practice Guideline #8.* Rockville, MD. U.S. Department of Health and Human Services.

VAHLENSIECK, W., AND G. RUTISHAUSER, EDS. 1992. *Benign Prostate Diseases.* New York. Thieme Medical Publishers.

Chapter 12

BRUSKEWITZ, R. 1992. "Benign Prostatic Hyperplasia: Drug and Nondrug Therapies." *Geriatrics.* 47(12): 39–45.

CHAPPLE, C. 1992. "Medical Treatment for Benign Prostatic Hyperplasia." *British Medical Journal.* 304(6836): 1198–1199.

KHOURY, S. 1992. "Future Directions in the Management of Benign Prostatic Hyperplasia." *British Journal of Urology.* 70(Suppl. 1): 27–32.

PETROVICH, Z. 1993. "New Trends in the Treatment of Benign Prostatic Hyperplasia and Carcinoma of the Prostate." *American Journal of Clinical Oncology.* 16(3): 187–200.

RAMSEY, E. 1993. "Transurethral Resection of the Prostate: Still the Gold Standard?" *Canadian Journal of Surgery.* 36(1): 9–10.

STONE, N. 1992. "Treatment Options in Benign Prostatic Hypertrophy." *Hospital Practice.* 27(10A): 85–92.

INDEX